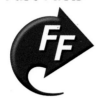

JAN -- 2012

W9-AVA-114

Fast Facts:
Eating Disorders

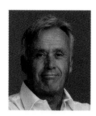

Hans Steiner MD

Professor of Psychiatry

Stanford University School of Medicine

Department of Psychiatry and Behavioral Sciences

Stanford, California, USA

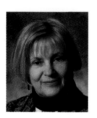

Martine F Flament MD PhD

Professor of Psychiatry and Psychology

Director, Youth Research Unit

University of Ottawa

Institute of Mental Health Research

Royal Ottawa Mental Health Centre

Ottawa, Ontario, Canada

Declaration of Independence

This book is as balanced and as practical as we can make it.

Ideas for improvement are always welcome: feedback@fastfacts.com

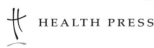
HEALTH PRESS

Fast Facts: Eating Disorders
First published January 2012

Text © 2012 Hans Steiner, Martine F Flament
© 2012 in this edition Health Press Limited
Health Press Limited, Elizabeth House, Queen Street, Abingdon,
Oxford OX14 3LN, UK
Tel: +44 (0)1235 523233
Fax: +44 (0)1235 523238

Book orders can be placed by telephone or via the website.
For regional distributors or to order via the website, please go to:
www.fastfacts.com
For telephone orders, please call +44 (0)1752 202301 (UK, Europe and Asia–Pacifiic),
1 800 247 6553 (USA, toll free) or +1 419 281 1802 (Americas).

Fast Facts is a trademark of Health Press Limited.

A CIP record for this title is available from the British Library.

ISBN 978-1-903734-91-9

Steiner H (Hans)
Fast Facts: Eating Disorders/
Hans Steiner, Martine F Flament

Typesetting and page layout by Zed, Oxford, UK.
Printed by Latimer Trend & Company Limited, Plymouth, UK.

Text printed with vegetable inks on biodegradable and recyclable
paper manufactured using elemental chlorine free (ECF) wood
pulp from well-managed forests.

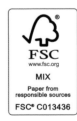

FSC
www.fsc.org
MIX
Paper from
responsible sources
FSC® C013436

Perspectives

Hans Steiner writes: This poem is a powerful glimpse of what the acute phase of these illnesses looks like from within. What comes through is tremendous disappointment and loneliness which needs combating before healing and forward-moving development can be restored. It is not clear who exactly the poet is referring to: parent, doctor, teacher, sister, aunt. But the message is clear: positive and powerful female role models in girls' lives are tremendously important and an essential part of recovery. The second perspective tells us that patients can, with support and effective treatment, find their point of 'balance'.

Persephone's Mother Pays a Visit
You dread this part: entering the room
where the child you slowly do not recognize
waits, all bone-shiver and whisper
of robes in the flickering dim.

She's losing it, she tells you.
Shedding when she runs her fingers through it.
Brittle as grass-husks under snow—

the girl has become nothing but a mouth,
closed to their pleas to open,
take and eat.

Witness to her waning pulse,
you greet her with a red-rimmed gaze,
those flowers she has grown to hate.
It's a matter of principle:

they're alive and she's not,
so she withers them with a glance,
and turns your hopes for antidotes to guilt
in what she doesn't say:

that you nurtured the earth
while she starved to death— no, *in* death already
this maiden of nothing, feasting on empty platters—

you grew the field that led her to her fall,
the food that trapped her there. Gave her hell
a start but not an end; sickness without cure.

The scene replays itself and each time,
you're helpless as she reaches for the seeds
of that ripe fruit. How they glisten, even in memory,
butcher-block red like the landscape of your heart

now, in the frailing light, as you leave her —
alone in the knowledge that you had a part in this,
that you were no mother to her,
only a goddess who failed.

Isabelle Fukutomi

"I have been an eating disorder patient for the last 21 years. For
many of these years my anorexia/bulimia was the most important
part of my life. In and out of the hospital, I became increasingly
isolated from my family and friends. My doctors and treatment
team became my social network. The transition back to normal
life was slow and erratic, but I am fortunate to have had the
patient and flexible medical and psychological care I needed.

I now have a family and have learned healthier, more productive
ways to create the order and structure once provided by my disease.
I still struggle with associated issues, but with my children as my
priority, I have managed to find a mostly successful balance."

A patient

Introduction

The classic eating disorders anorexia nervosa and bulimia nervosa represent relatively common and significant disturbances that are now being seen with increasing frequency by healthcare professionals. Within the carefully coordinated and comprehensive multidisciplinary intervention that is required for every patient with an eating disorder, the primary care team has an important role in initial screening and in the subsequent monitoring of the patient's physical state. There is evidence that treatment can be successful; however, it is unclear if significant risks and vulnerabilities for recurrence ever completely resolve.

Eating disorders are classic 'psychosomatic' syndromes in the sense that psychological and somatic functioning are inextricably intertwined. In *Fast Facts: Eating Disorders*, we look at the association between pathological thoughts and emotions concerning appearance, eating and food. We also examine the deviant eating behavior that can lead to alterations in body composition and functioning.

Eating disorders are often conceptualized as developmental disorders. However, few prospective studies have examined normative and pathological phenomena in populations at risk. Only a few studies have employed longitudinal designs, and these are discussed where appropriate throughout the book.

This book summarizes the available evidence base that underpins the current diagnosis and treatment for eating disorders, which we have broadly divided into anorexia, bulimia and related disorders. We discuss in some detail the role of the primary care physician in identifying the disorder, working with the treatment team and providing essential therapeutic services.

Classification

Definition of anorexia nervosa

Anorexia nervosa is characterized by the refusal to maintain a bodyweight equal to or above a minimally normal weight for the individual's age and height. Bodyweight is at least 15% below the norm. The weight loss is self-induced by several means:

- fasting
- use of laxatives or diuretics
- self-induced vomiting
- excessive exercise.

Individuals with anorexia exhibit an overwhelming fear of putting on weight and a distorted view of the size and shape of their body. Postmenarcheal females experience amenorrhea, i.e. the absence of at least three consecutive menstrual cycles, or if the menstrual cycle occurs it does so only as a result of hormone administration.

There are two subtypes of anorexia:

- restricting type, in which the individual does not regularly engage in binge-eating or purging behavior
- binge-eating/purging type, in which the individual regularly engages in binge-eating or purging behavior.

Binge-eating is characterized by eating large amounts of food in a discrete amount of time and feeling a sense of a lack of control. Purging behavior includes self-induced vomiting or the misuse of laxatives, diuretics or enemas.

The specific diagnostic criteria for anorexia from the fourth edition of the American Psychiatric Association's *Diagnostic and Statistical Manual of Mental Disorders* (DSM-IV) are discussed in more detail in Chapter 4 – Diagnosis.

Definition of bulimia nervosa

Bulimia nervosa is characterized by recurrent episodes of significant binge-eating – eating large amounts of food in a discrete amount of time and feeling a sense of a lack of control – followed by inappropriate compensatory behaviors to prevent weight gain. There are two subtypes of bulimia:

- purging type, in which the individual regularly engages in purging behavior, such as self-induced vomiting or the misuse of laxatives, diuretics or enemas
- non-purging type, in which the individual does not regularly engage in purging behavior, but uses other inappropriate compensatory behaviors such as fasting or excessive exercising.

Those who suffer from bulimia use their binge and purge cycles to prevent weight gain and to regulate other emotional difficulties. Unlike anorexia, bulimia does not generally result in significant weight loss and in many ways is a very secretive disease. The shame and isolation experienced by individuals suffering from this disorder can hinder recovery.

The specific DSM-IV diagnostic criteria for bulimia are discussed in more detail in Chapter 4 – Diagnosis.

Definition of eating disorders not otherwise specified

DSM-IV classifies both anorexia and bulimia under a specific diagnostic category entitled 'Eating Disorders', which also includes a third classification entitled 'eating disorders not otherwise specified' ('atypical eating disorder' in the World Health Organization's *International Statistical Classification of Diseases and Related Health Problems*, tenth revision [ICD-10]). This last category includes binge-eating disorder and night-eating syndrome, discussed in Chapter 9 of this book, and may be used to describe eating disorders that meet some but not all of the diagnostic criteria for anorexia or bulimia: for example, an individual with almost all of the symptoms of anorexia but who still has a normal and regular menstrual cycle and/or a normal body mass index, or cases with overevaluation of weight and shape associated with purging behaviors at least twice a week but no binge-eating episodes ('eating disorder not otherwise specified' [EDNOS] purging type). Patients that present with subsyndromal criteria should be monitored in order to identify the development of a full-syndrome eating disorder. Primary care physicians should conduct a comprehensive assessment to uncover any significant risk factors in the patient's life that could rapidly lead to a full-syndrome eating disorder. The primary care physician may invite the patient for serial assessments to track symptoms over time, consulting or referring with a specialist if needed.

Key points – classification

- Anorexia nervosa is characterized by the refusal to maintain a normal bodyweight by self-starvation.
- Bulimia nervosa is characterized by significant binge-eating and subsequent purging to control bodyweight.
- Eating disorders often remain secret; sufferers experience shame and isolation, which can hinder recovery.
- Other eating disorders include binge-eating disorder and night-eating syndrome.

Key references

APA. Eating disorders. *Diagnostic and Statistical Manual of Mental Disorders*, 4th edn. Text Revision (DSM-IV-TR). Washington, DC: American Psychiatric Association, 2000:589–94.

APA. *Practice Guidelines for the Treatment of Psychiatric Disorders, Compendium 2006; Eating Disorders*, 3rd edn. Washington, DC: American Psychiatric Association, May 2006.

Fairburn CG, Cooper Z, Bohn K et al. The severity and status of eating disorder NOS: implications for DSM-V. *Behav Res Ther* 2007;45: 1705–15.

WHO. ICD-10 *Classification of Mental and Behavioural Disorders*. Geneva: World Health Organization, 1993.

The most recent epidemiological studies on eating disorders are population based, specifically assess juveniles and use state-of-the-art two-stage screening designs that comprise surveys followed by interviews.

Anorexia

Published studies evaluating the incidence of anorexia (i.e. the number of new cases in a population over a specific period) have produced disparate results because of wide variations in the sampled geographical area, the methods used and the sources of case detection (e.g. inpatient or outpatient cases, public health services and/or private doctors, diagnostic criteria, content of medical files). The highest age-adjusted and sex-adjusted incidence rate was 8.3 per 100 000 person-years in Rochester, Minnesota, USA, using an extensive case-finding approach during the period of 1935–1989.

Sex differences. Eating disorders are far more prevalent among women. The UK's Royal College of Psychiatrists states that girls and women are ten times more likely than boys and men to suffer from anorexia. In the Rochester study the overall annual age-adjusted incidence was 14.6 women per 100 000 inhabitants. For men, the overall age-adjusted incidence was 1.8 per 100 000 inhabitants.

Age groups affected. In the same study in Rochester, 69.4 in 100 000 15–19 year-old girls had anorexia, which made it the third most frequent disorder among teenage girls in the USA. Time analyses showed that the incidence of anorexia in women decreased from 16.6 per 100 000 person-years in 1935–1939 to 7 per 100 000 in 1950–1954, but then increased to 26.3 per 100 000 in 1980–1984. Higher rates mirrored times in history in which the media portrayed thinner models, actors and celebrities. The more severe and unremitting form of anorexia may have remained constant, but teenagers – being more vulnerable to cultural pressures – will have been more likely to develop a milder form of the illness in response to such pressures. In Europe, the incidence of anorexia seems to have been rather stable since 1970.

The prevalence (total number of cases in a population at a specific point or over a given period) of anorexia within secondary-education establishments has been studied in the USA, Great Britain, Sweden, Switzerland, Italy, Spain, Portugal and Australia. Studies of at least 1000 girls and young women (aged 10–23 years), including face-to-face interviews, have shown the overall prevalence of anorexia to range from 0.1% to 0.9%. Among adult women, the lifetime prevalence of anorexia ranges from 0.3% according to a narrow clinical definition to 3.7% according to a broad clinical definition. In a meta-analysis, the 1-year prevalence rate of anorexia in the community was calculated as 0.37% in young females.

The peak age of onset of anorexia is between 13 and 15 years of age. Thus prevalence and incidence are particularly high among 15–25-year-olds, who constitute approximately 40% of all identified cases (Figure 2.1).

Prepubescent onset (before menarche) is rare but further study of this age group is needed. Personality characteristics and eating disorder psychopathology are unique in this population and the course of the disorder in this group is particularly severe.

Ethnic differences. Anorexia has long been considered as a disorder affecting mainly young women from middle to high economic classes in wealthy countries. While the disorder continues to be more prevalent in Western industrialized nations of white ethnicity and in middle- to upper-class women, there is an increasing diversity of those affected in terms of socioeconomic status and ethnicity, including African, Asian and Indian groups.

In the USA, significant differences in the prevalence of anorexia were found by race in a geographically and economically diverse community sample of white and black 19–24-year-old women; none of the black women was found to have had anorexia (Figure 2.2).

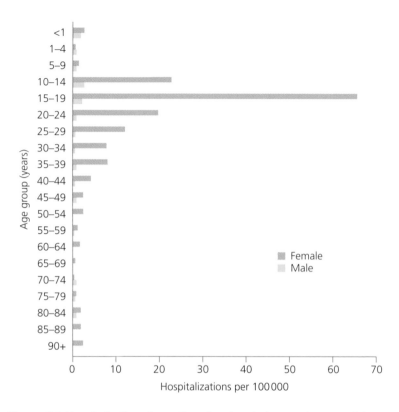

Figure 2.1 Hospitalizations for eating disorders (using most responsible diagnosis only) in general hospitals per 100 000 by age group, Canada 1999/2000. Reproduced with permission from Center for Chronic Disease Prevention and Control, Health Canada, using data from Hospital Morbidity File, Canadian Institute for Health Information.

Bulimia

Only a few incidence studies of bulimia have been conducted, with an annual incidence rate of 13.5 per 100 000 person-years in Rochester, USA, and 6.6 per 100 000 person-years in the UK.

Sex differences. As with other eating disorders, bulimia has a much higher prevalence in women than in men. The reported lifetime prevalence of bulimia ranges from 1.0% to 2.8% among women, and is about 0.5% among men. In France, a two-stage screening for bulimia

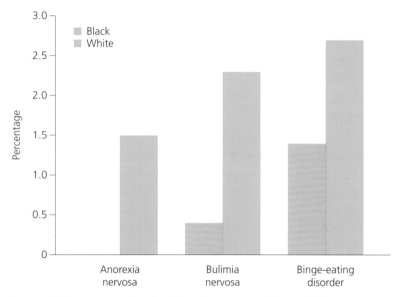

Figure 2.2 Prevalence of eating disorders among white and black women in the USA, 2003. Adapted from data in Striegel-Moore RH et al. 2003.

among 3527 unselected secondary-school students demonstrated higher rates in girls than boys with regard to overconcern with bodyweight and shape, dieting, bulimic binges, self-induced vomiting, use of laxatives and use of diet pills. From these data the researchers estimated prevalences for bulimia of approximately 1.1% in girls and 0.2% in boys.

The male to female prevalence ratio for bulimia is 1:5. However, the disorder may be increasingly affecting male athletes and performers. Only a very small minority of female and male individuals with bulimia in the community enter the mental healthcare system.

Age groups affected. The peak age of onset for bulimia is in late adolescence or early adulthood, between 17 and 25 years of age. The condition is less frequently found in teenagers than in adult women.

Ethnic differences. Bulimia is more commonly found in Western industrialized nations, specifically in populations that are of middle- and upper-class socioeconomic status. Nevertheless, in the past decade, populations of young African, Latino and Asian women have also been adversely affected as bulimia has reached more diverse populations. In the US community sample of women aged 19–24 years of age described above, the odds of detecting bulimia in white women were six times that of black women (see Figure 2.2).

Other eating disorders

Epidemiological studies show that even in individuals who do not match the criteria for a specific eating disorder, patterns of 'disordered eating' are highly prevalent. 'Eating disorders not otherwise specified' (EDNOS; see page 10) are probably more common than classic eating disorders in young people.

In the USA, the Centers for Disease Control and Prevention's 2005 Youth Risk Behavior Survey found that 30% of boys and 62% of girls in high school were trying to lose weight, although only 25% of boys and 38% of girls considered themselves to be overweight. Adolescents employ unhealthy weight control behaviors such as fasting (12%), diet supplements (6%) and even purging by vomiting or laxative abuse (5%). In both adolescents and adults, atypical eating disorders (EDNOS) account for more than 50% of cases in the community and in eating disorder treatment clinics.

Key points – epidemiology

- Eating disorders are more common in women than men, but disordered eating is increasingly being seen in male athletes and performers.
- Both anorexia and bulimia are more prevalent in Western industrialized nations of white ethnicity and in middle- to upper-class women, but the disorders are now affecting more diverse populations in terms of ethnicity and socioeconomic status.
- Bulimia is more common in adults than teenagers, while anorexia is more common in adolescent girls.
- Disordered eating is probably more common than classic eating disorders in adolescents and young adults.

Key references

American Medical Association. *Eating Disorders and Promotion of Healthy Body Image. Report 8 of the Council on Science and Public Health (A-07)*. American Medical Association, 2007.

Arnow B, Sanders MJ, Steiner H. Premenarcheal versus postmenarcheal anorexia nervosa: a comparative study. *Clin Child Psychol Psychiatry* 1999;4:3:403–14.

Flament M, Ledoux S, Jeammet P et al. A population study of bulimia nervosa and subclinical eating disorders in adolescence. In: Steinhausen HC, ed. *Eating Disorders in Adolescence: Anorexia and Bulimia Nervosa*. New York: Walter de Gruyter, 1995;21–36.

Garfinkel PE, Lin E, Goering P et al. Bulimia nervosa in a Canadian community sample: prevalence and comparison of subgroups. *Am J Psychiatry* 1995;152:1052–8.

Hoek HW. Incidence, prevalence and mortality of anorexia nervosa and other eating disorders. *Current Opin Psychiatry* 2006;19:389–94.

Hoek HW, van Hoeken D. Review of the prevalence and incidence of eating disorders. *Int J Eat Disord* 2003;34:383–96.

Hudson JI, Hiripi E, Pope HG, Jr., Kessler RC. The prevalence and correlates of eating disorders in the National Comorbidity Survey Replication. *Biol Psychiatry* 2007;61:348–58.

Kalm LM, Semba RD. They starved so that others be better fed: remembering Ancel Keys and the Minnesota experiment. *J Nutr* 2005;135:1347–52.

Keel PK, Klump KL. Are eating disorders culture-bound syndromes? Implications for conceptualizing their etiology. *Psychol Bull* 2003;129:747–69.

Lucas AR, Beard CM, O'Fallon WM, Kurland LT. 50-year trends in the incidence of anorexia nervosa in Rochester, Minn.: a population-based study. *Am J Psychiatry* 1991;148:917–22.

Striegel-Moore RH, Dohm FA, Kraemer HC et al. Eating disorders in white and black women. *Am J Psychiatry* 2003;160:1326–31.

Walters EE, Kendler KS. Anorexia nervosa and anorexic-like syndromes in a population-based female twin sample. *Am J Psychiatry* 1995;152:64–71.

The origins of eating disorders are widely seen as a complex combination of biological and environmental factors. Various genetic, developmental, psychological, familial and social variables have been suggested as risk factors.

Biological factors

Genetic factors. The current state of the genetics of eating disorders is that while there is familial clustering of these syndromes, it is not at all clear that they are in their entirety genetically transmitted disorders. Whatever the genetic component to each one of them, it seems to be stronger for anorexia than bulimia. And granting even that, the current literature supports a polygenetic transmission of risk which needs substantial accumulation of environmental risk to have disorders come to the fore.

The most potent risk factor for eating disorders is female gender (see Chapter 2). This association is likely to reflect biological as well as psychosocial factors.

Family studies indicate that first-degree relatives of patients with anorexia have an increased prevalence of eating disorders (Table 3.1), and that first-degree relatives of patients with bulimia or binge-eating disorder appear to be at increased risk of eating disorders, mood disorders and substance abuse. Twin studies of anorexia and bulimia suggest there is approximately a 50–80% genetic contribution to liability accounted for by additive genetic factors.

Candidate gene studies have initially focused on the serotonergic and other neurotransmitter system genes involved in bodyweight regulation, with hardly any unequivocally confirmed findings. Systematic genome-wide linkage scans based on families with at least two individuals with an eating disorder revealed initial linkage regions on chromosomes 1, 3, 4 (anorexia) and 10p (bulimia). Ongoing international collaborations are working at pooling cases and using newer forms of analysis such as genome-wide associations.

TABLE 3.1

Prevalence of eating disorders according to familial relationship

Relationship to index case	Prevalence (%)
First-degree relative	29
Mother	27
Father	16
Sibling	3–10

Adapted from Steinhausen HC. Treatment and outcome of adolescent anorexia nervosa. *Horm Res* 1995;43:168–70.

Similar to other complex disorders, the eating disorders are likely to have a polygenic etiology, each gene having a relatively small effect.

Physiological factors. Both high and low premorbid body mass index (BMI) may predispose to anorexia. Being overweight or obese (with a high BMI) is a risk factor because of the likelihood of dieting, while low BMI may characterize individuals who are already prodromally ill with anorexia but who have not yet reached the weight criteria for definitive diagnosis.

Childhood obesity is a risk factor for bulimia and binge-eating disorder. A pear-shaped body and relatively high amounts of body fat may also predispose to eating disorders. People with one or both of these characteristics may have fat deposits that are hard to move by normal dieting; this may lead to the adoption of extreme weight-control measures.

Hormonal and neurohormonal influences. The study of the neurobiology of eating disorders has demonstrated large hormonal and neurohormonal differences in adult and late-adolescent patients who are acutely ill. Levels of histidyl-proline diketopiperazine, a hormone that is involved in the induction of satiety, are shown to increase as individuals with anorexia gain weight. This hormonal change may be responsible for premature feelings of satiation.

Around 20% of individuals with diabetes mellitus develop an eating disorder. Patients with type 1 diabetes are more likely to develop anorexia or bulimia, while patients with type 2 diabetes are more likely to develop binge-eating disorder. This suggests that insulin–glucagon systems may be involved in the predisposition for eating disorders. In addition, because energy requirements for weight rehabilitation and maintenance have been shown to differ in anorexic patients, bulimic patients and control populations, it is possible that premorbid metabolic abnormalities act as risk factors for eating disorders.

Neurobiological factors. Although many of the biological findings in eating disorders can be best understood as results of starvation and disturbed eating behaviors, some are causally linked as risk or maintaining factors. Considerable evidence suggests that altered brain serotonin function contributes to dysregulation of appetite, mood, and impulse control in eating disorders.

Dysregulation of the serotonergic system is usually secondary to weight changes. Studies have suggested that diminished serotonin activity may trigger some of the cognitive and mood disturbances associated with bulimia. The findings also indicated that chronic depletion of plasma tryptophan may be one of the mechanisms whereby persistent dieting can lead to the development of eating disorders in vulnerable individuals.

Brain monoamine function in eating disorders has been studied in both the acute state and after recovery, using specific ligands and positron emission tomography. There is a reduction in 5-HT_{2A} receptors and an increase in 5-HT_{1A} receptors in both the acute and recovered state, and dopamine receptors (DA_2) within the striatum are increased after recovery. Anomalies in the dopamine system could heighten food reward in bulimia and binge-eating disorder.

Abnormalities in both illness-related (food and body shape) and non-illness-related information processing have been detected with functional brain imaging studies. These functional abnormalities could maintain some of the eating disorder behaviors.

Environmental factors

Family functioning. Historically, the role of dysfunctional styles of family interaction was put forward in theories of the development of eating disorders. Unfortunately and unfairly, this has led to some parenting styles being blamed for causing eating disorders in children. Still, the type of relationships that children and adolescents develop with food and body image, both healthy and unhealthy, is strongly influenced by:

- parental attitudes toward eating, weight and body shape
- parental eating and weight-related behavior modeled in the home
- excessive parental control over a child's nutritional intake such that the child is unable to make independent food choices.

Perceived pressure to be thin, family criticism regarding weight, and maternal investment in slenderness predict eating disturbances in adolescents. Parents also have a strong influence over their children's internalization of the aesthetic ideal.

Anorexia. When compared with control families, those with an anorexic child tend to show more rigid organization, less clear interpersonal boundaries, and avoidance of open discussion of disagreements between parents and children. Patients with an eating disorder seem to be more likely than controls to experience attachment disturbances, such as insecure and anxious attachment styles and deactivating defensive strategies. Furthermore, families of individuals with anorexia tend to have a higher rate of parental eating disorders, family dieting and adverse comments from family members about eating, weight or appearance.

Bulimia. The families of individuals with bulimia are often more chaotic and conflicted. These families tend to have higher rates of alcoholism, substance misuse and affective disorders, as well as higher levels of perfectionism and a sense of ineffectiveness.

Societal influences. The preoccupation with body image and the drive to attain thinness that are characteristic of eating disorders relate to the idealized representation of the human figure within a given culture, and to the pressure to conform from peers and the media. In Western countries, the body dimensions of female cultural icons, such as fashion models and actresses, have become progressively thinner over the past decades, with a concomitant rise in disordered eating among women. Mounting evidence implicates the mass media in the promotion of body-image and eating disturbances, with the emphasis on dieting and other weight-control behaviors often targeted at women rather than men, thus paralleling the gender distribution of eating pathology. A longitudinal prospective study of ethnic Fijian adolescent girls demonstrated an increase in key indicators of disordered eating following novel prolonged television exposure to the aesthetic ideal.

The internalization of societal pressures has been shown to have a clear effect on body dissatisfaction and eating dysregulation in population samples. The first diet in adolescent girls is most frequently triggered by comparison with others' appearance and their own self-ideal. Societal influences and internalization of the thin ideal may lead directly to body dissatisfaction and unhealthy eating, or may be mediated by more general psychological processes such as intrapersonal (self-esteem, mood, personality) or interpersonal functioning and/or emotional regulation and coping.

Stressors and life events precipitate the onset of eating disorders in 70% of cases, and include parental neglect, abuse, indifference, loss and separation. In some studies, a high incidence of sexual abuse during childhood is reported by women with diagnosed eating disorders; rates of abuse are seemingly higher in bulimia than anorexia. In a US statewide representative sample, both sexual and physical abuse were strong independent risk factors for disordered eating in adolescent girls and boys. The nature of this relationship is difficult to assess because of differences in diagnostic criteria for abuse, a high base rate of sexual abuse in the general female population and a high rate of abuse associated with other psychiatric diagnoses. The issue is insufficiently explored in young people. Male university students who reported physical and sexual abuse in childhood were also at a greater risk for eating disorders.

A wide range of other childhood adversities and stressful life events has been associated with eating problems during adolescence. In one large referred population of patients with eating disorders, 55% reported recent stressful life events, most often separation (e.g. death of an important other, parental divorce, separation from close ones) or other changes in family or living conditions.

The effects of stress on eating are not uniform. Stress-induced hyperphagia (an abnormally increased appetite for, and consumption of, food) occurs more often in children and adults who are dietary-restrained eaters than in those who are not. Thus, for the vast majority of children and adults, the effects of current stress on food intake seem to be moderated by intermittent dietary restraint.

Developmental factors

Life-stage risk factors have been identified at the major developmental phases of childhood and adolescence.

Preschool. It is still debatable whether there is a correlation between eating problems in early childhood and those in adolescence. The demographics of early feeding problems suggest no association, because boys are more likely to exhibit disordered eating in early childhood, whereas girls are at greater risk in adolescence. However, early childhood feeding and eating problems, such as pica, picky eating, digestive problems, as well as eating conflicts, struggles around meals, and unpleasant meals, have been found to predict eating disorders in adolescence or young adulthood. Mothers of patients with eating disorders have reported reliance on scheduled feeding and prematurely introduced solids more frequently than controls. However, these practices were also used with siblings who did not become ill, suggesting that other factors are likely to be involved in the pathogenesis of eating disorders.

In one study, six eating behaviors were evaluated at three time points over 2.5 years by maternal interview in two different overlapping cohorts (aged 0–10 and 9–18 years). Early maladaptive eating patterns were associated with a greater likelihood of problems later in life. Picky eating and digestive problems predicted preanorexic behavior. Early eating problems were also a predictor of the future onset of bulimia.

School-age children. In elementary school (7–12 years), significant numbers of children want to be thinner than they are. Studies indicate that 37% try some form of weight loss, and 6.9% score in the pathological range on an adapted version of the Eating Attitudes Test (see Table 4.8, page 46). There are few significant differences between boys and girls. Body-image distortions in this age group are associated with dieting and weight concerns. Food refusal, ritualistic behavior during meals, phobic behavior and elevated internalizing behaviors such as depression and anxiety have all been described in school-age children who eventually suffer from an eating disorder.

Prepuberty and adolescence. Studies have also confirmed that eating problems emerge in response to pubertal change, especially fat accumulation. Girls who feel most negatively about their bodies at puberty are at a higher risk of developing eating difficulties. Several studies have identified associations between disturbed eating in adolescents and:
- anxious attachment
- weight concerns
- deficient self-regulation
- affective lability
- concerns about current body shape.

Contextual risk factors during this developmental phase include:
- teasing by peers
- discomfort about discussing problems with parents
- maternal preoccupation with diets
- acculturation to Western values in immigrants.

First-generation immigrants, for example, are less likely to develop anorexia than the second and later generations.

Interestingly, homosexual boys (12–20 years) have a far greater frequency of disordered eating and weight concerns than heterosexual boys, for complex reasons that are currently not well understood.

Anorexia seems to occur at a precise timepoint in adolescent development, possibly reflecting the young person's inability to manage the developmental demands of adolescence. Adolescence is also a time marked by an increase in fat deposition for girls, and an unease and unhappiness with bodily appearance. In a sample of 808 girls (12–14 years) with no clinical symptoms, 34% stated a strong desire to lose weight; of these, 34% had a body mass index (BMI) of less than 20 (i.e. in the normal or thin range). Furthermore, 24% restricted their food intake to influence their weight and shape, 5% engaged in 8-hour fasting for more than half of each week and 38% undertook vigorous exercise to control their weight.

The biological changes of puberty certainly contribute to the onset of eating disorders. In girls, the peripubertal rise in estrogens affects mood and appetite regulation, because estrogens modulate serotonergic function via a variety of mechanisms, including changes in serotonin receptor number, serotonin synthesis and metabolism. Interestingly, dieting, a common factor that precipitates binge-eating behavior, alters brain serotonin function more markedly in women than in men. Estrogens also enhance stress responsiveness through downregulation of the hypothalamo–pituitary–adrenocortical axis.

In girls, an association between early pubertal timing and eating-disorder symptoms as well as diagnosis has been observed in a number of studies.

Individual variables

Intrapersonal factors. Affective disturbances have been proposed as underlying disorders for bulimia, and a similar relationship has been proposed between anorexia and obsessive–compulsive disorders.

Depression is one of the most salient psychiatric comorbidities in both men and women with eating disorders. Dysregulation in serotonin, a neurotransmitter involved in the regulation of both mood and satiety, has been implicated as a causal factor in depression and eating disorders. Antidepressants that selectively block serotonin reuptake are effective in the treatment of both depression and bulimia or binge-eating disorder.

Anxiety and obsessive–compulsive behavior. Similarly, increased levels of anxiety and obsessiveness have been described in young people and adults with eating disorders. Premorbid overanxious disorder and obsessive–compulsive tendencies are seen significantly more often in patients with anorexia than in controls.

Similarly, the risk for bulimia is increased by the presence of overanxious disorder or social phobia relative to controls. However, longitudinal studies in other fields indicate that premorbid anxiety disorders and negative affectivity are also risk factors for the development of other psychiatric conditions such as affective disorders and substance abuse.

Anger. Clinicians have described internalized anger and rage as primary emotions in patients with eating disorders. Researchers have found higher levels of perceived external control, lower assertiveness, lower self-esteem and more self-directed hostility in individuals with anorexia and bulimia than in controls.

Body-image disturbance is a well-known risk factor for clinical and subclinical levels of eating disorders. It has been related to indices of global psychological functioning, such as self-esteem, anxiety, depression and negative affectivity. However, body-image disturbance seems to be more closely related to restricted eating, and global psychological functioning more closely related to bulimia.

Body dissatisfaction is not only a defining characteristic of eating disorders but also a contributing factor in their development and maintenance. The unhealthy weight-control behaviors that characterize eating disorders, such as strict dieting, excessive exercise or laxative/diuretic abuse, are used to compensate for negative perceptions of body size, shape or weight. In a Canadian study of middle-school adolescents (early teens), negative perception of physical appearance and high importance of social acceptance correlated significantly with high levels of disordered eating.

Personality traits. Girls and women with anorexia tend to be anxious, inhibited and controlled, while those with bulimia tend to be more affectively labile and impulsive.

Negative self-evaluation, perfectionism and obsessive–compulsive behavior are all psychological traits that promote dieting behavior and are more commonly found in those with anorexia than in those with other psychiatric disturbances. A desire to avoid conflict predisposes the anorexic to focus on the more easily controllable domain of the body and weight. Being a perfectionist and a self-disciplinarian allows a person to maintain the strict diet and exercise regimen necessary for the sustainment of the disorder.

Psychological risk factors associated with bulimia include negative self-evaluation, shyness, a lack of close friends, missing school, perfectionism and mood lability.

Interpersonal functioning. Girls have been described as different from boys in their self-perceptions, emotions and behaviors pertaining to interpersonal relationships. Numerous studies have been conducted on the influence of peers on eating behavior and body image. Pressure to be thin from friends or weight-based teasing from peers has been associated with subclinical eating disturbances in high-school girls and with full-blown eating disorders in college-age women. Negative social feedback, in the form of teasing a person about their appearance, has been indicated as a possible etiologic factor in the development of disordered eating.

Impulse behaviors and substance abuse. Bulimic patients have a history of impulsive behaviors, including alcohol and drug misuse, suicidal behaviors and shoplifting. These problematic behaviors are often overlooked on initial contact. The preoccupation with food often impairs patients' functioning in social-, school- and work-related activities. The pattern of impulsive behaviors associated with bulimia is not common in those with anorexia.

A review of the literature on the comorbidity of eating disorders and substance abuse reveals an association between the two, especially among bulimics.

- 17% of bulimics report a current or past history of drug, substance or alcohol abuse and/or dependence, or treatment for any of the above.
- 20% of drug abusers report a current or past history of bulimia or bulimic behaviors.
- Among bulimics, the family history studies show alcoholism rates of 39%, and drug or substance use rates of 19%.

When treating a patient with either an eating disorder or a substance-abuse problem, the clinician should always consider the possibility of a comorbid substance-abuse or eating problem.

Several psychological and biological mechanisms have been proposed to explain the comorbidity of eating disorders and substance abuse.

Psychological factors include the hypothesis of an addictive personality that predisposes individuals to becoming addicted to substances, viewing food and drugs as functional equivalents. Another explanation, which has received empirical support, is that the initial development of an addiction fosters psychological and behavioral patterns that enable individuals to develop other addictions. Another mechanism is the self-medication hypothesis, which states that individuals with an eating disorder turn to alcohol and drugs in order to cope with, or treat, their eating problems. The same has been said about depression – afflicted individuals turn to food or drugs to treat their depression.

Biological factors have been investigated in terms of the genetic contributions to alcoholism, drug abuse and eating disorders. Similarities in the process of these disorders suggest biological mechanisms underlying the addiction.

Key points – etiology and pathogenesis

- Clinicians and patients are best served by considering eating disorders from a bio-psycho-social perspective, unified in a framework of developmental psychopathology. All components are present, and interact to increase the risk for disorder as development proceeds. Disorder represents the crystallization of these interactions into syndromes which, in this case, are a developmental outcome, not simply the burgeoning of a latent biological deficit, as reductionist models of psychopathology would have it.
- Eating problems usually emerge in the context of pubertal change.
- Parental attitudes and behaviors towards eating, weight and body shape have a strong influence on the development of a child's relationship with food and body image, both healthy and unhealthy.
- Stressors and life events, such as childhood abuse, separations or bereavement, may precipitate the onset of eating disorders.
- Psychiatric comorbidities in both men and women with eating disorders include depression, anxiety, obsessive behavior and body-image disturbance.
- When treating a patient with either an eating disorder or substance-abuse problem, clinicians should always consider the possibility of comorbidity.

Key references

Agras S, Hammer L, McNicholas F. A prospective study of the influence of eating-disordered mothers on their children. *Int J Eat Disord* 1999;25:253–62.

Becker AE, Burwell RA, Gilman SE et al. Eating behaviors and attitudes following prolonged exposure to television among ethnic Fijian adolescent girls. *Br J Psychiatry* 2002;180:509–14.

Fairburn CG, Brownell KD. *Eating Disorders and Obesity: A Comprehensive Handbook*, 2nd edn. New York: Guilford Press, 2002.

Flament M, Bissada H, Spettigue W. Evidence-based pharmacotherapy of eating disorders. *Int J Neuropsychopharmacol*, 2011. Epub ahead of print (doi: 10.1017/S1461145711000381).

Godart NT, Flament MF, Perdereau F, Jeammet P. Comorbidity between eating disorders and anxiety disorders: a review. *Int J Eat Disord* 2002;32:253–70.

Jacobi C, Hayward C, de Zwaan M et al. Coming to terms with risk factors for eating disorders: application of risk terminology and suggestions for a general taxonomy. *Psychol Bull* 2004;130:19–65.

Johnson JG, Cohen P, Kasen S, Brook JS. Childhood adversities associated with risk for eating disorders or weight problems during adolescence or early childhood. *Am J Psychiatry* 2002;159:394–400.

Kaye W. Neurobiology of anorexia and bulimia nervosa. *Physiol Behav* 2008;94:121–35.

Keel PK, Klump KL. Are eating disorders culture-bound syndromes? Implications for conceptualizing their etiology. *Psychol Bull* 2003;129:747–69.

Mazzeo SE, Mitchell KS, Bulik CM et al. Assessing the heritability of anorexia nervosa symptoms using a marginal maximal likelihood approach. *Psychol Med* 2009;39:463–73.

Mazzeo SE, Mitchell KS, Bulik CM et al. A twin study of specific bulimia nervosa symptoms. *Psychol Med* 2010;40:1203–13.

McVey GL, Pepler D, Davis R et al. Risk and protective factors associated with disordered eating during early adolescence. *J Early Adolesc* 2002;22:75–95.

Mitchell KS, Neale MC, Bulik CM et al. Binge eating disorder: a symptom-level investigation of genetic and environmental influences on liability. *Psychol Med* 2010;40:1899–906.

Scherag S, Hebebrand J, Hinney A. Eating disorders: the current status of molecular genetic research. *Eur Child Adolesc Psychiatry* 2010;19:211–26.

Steiger H. Eating disorders and the serotonin connection: state, trait and developmental effects. *J Psychiatry Neurosci* 2004;29:20–9.

Steiner H, ed. *Handbook of Developmental Psychiatry: Children and Adolescents*. Hackensack: World Scientific Publishing, 2011.

Steiner H, Lock J. Anorexia nervosa and bulimia nervosa in children and adolescents: a review of the past 10 years. *J Am Acad Child Adolesc Psychiatry* 1998;37:352–9.

Ward A, Ramsay R, Turnbull S et al. Attachment in anorexia nervosa: a transgenerational perspective. *Br J Med Psychol* 2001;74:497–505.

Active screening for eating disorders is a reasonable practice, as they are common in adolescents, particularly in high-risk groups such as athletes, performing artists, models and actors.

In most cases of anorexia nervosa, parents bring in their child for a medical evaluation. Girls may be brought to the family practitioner or gynecologist because of menstrual irregularity. Because they are brought to see the physician, as opposed to voluntarily seeking help, the adolescent may be in a state of denial. It is therefore important to question both the patient and the parents. The denial can make assessment difficult, so more than one visit may be necessary to uncover all the information needed. Additionally, clinical assessment over time is important to better understand the nature of the patient's symptoms and to develop an appropriate treatment approach. In contrast, individuals with bulimia or binge-eating disorder typically come on their own, and might not wish to disclose their concerns and disturbed eating behaviors to their parents or significant others.

The clinical assessment should consist of a medical history, family history, physical examination and laboratory testing. Questions to ask the patient and parents to aid diagnosis are listed in Table 4.1.

Diagnostic criteria

The American Psychiatric Association's *Diagnostic and Statistical Manual of Mental Disorders*, fourth edition, (DSM-IV) criteria for anorexia and bulimia are highlighted in Tables 4.2 and 4.3, respectively. In the alternative diagnostic classification used in Europe – the World Health Organization's *International Statistical Classification of Diseases and Related Health Problems*, tenth revision (ICD-10) – eating disorders belong to a wider category entitled 'Behavioral syndromes associated with physiological disturbances and physical factors'. The ICD-10 criteria for anorexia and bulimia are consistent with those of DSM-IV, the only significant difference being the relationship between bulimia and anorexia. DSM-IV gives precedence to anorexia over bulimia, while

TABLE 4.1

Screening questions for the diagnosis of eating disorders

Key screening questions

How much would you like to weigh?

How do you feel about your present weight?

Do you or anyone else have any concerns about your eating or exercise behaviors/practices?

Detailed screening questions

History of present illness

- What has been your maximum weight and when?
- How frequently do you weigh yourself?
- When did you begin to lose weight?
- What weight-control methods have you tried?

Diet history

- What are your current dietary practices? Ask for specifics, amounts, food groups, fluids, restrictions
- Do you binge eat? Find out frequency, amount, triggers
- Do you purge/vomit after eating? Find out frequency, amount, triggers and how long after meals
- Do you use any diuretics, laxatives, diet pills, ipecac syrup (causes vomiting)?

Exercise

- What exercise do you currently take? Find out details of types, frequency, duration, intensity
- How stressed are you if you miss a workout?

Menstrual history

- When did you have your first menstrual period?
- How regular are your menstrual cycles?
- When was your last normal menstrual period?

CONTINUED

TABLE 4.1 (CONTINUED)

Review symptoms

- Do you experience any of the following?
  - dizziness, blackouts, weakness, fatigue
  - pallor, easy bruising or bleeding
  - cold intolerance
  - hair loss, lanugo, dry skin
  - vomiting, diarrhea, constipation
  - fullness, bloating, abdominal pain, epigastric burning
  - muscle cramps, joint pains, palpitations, chest pain
  - menstrual irregularities
- Also assess:
  - symptoms of hyperthyroidism, diabetes, malignancy, infection, inflammatory bowel disease
  - psychological symptoms/history
  - adjustment to pubertal development
  - body image/self-esteem
  - anxiety, depression, obsessive–compulsive disorder, other psychiatric conditions

Past medical history

- Is there a family history of obesity, eating disorders, depression, other mental illness, substance abuse/alcoholism?

Social history

- Gain details of home environment, school environment, activities, substance use, sexual history, physical or sexual abuse

From American Medical Association. *Report 8 of the Council on Science and Public Health (A-07). Eating Disorders and Promotion of Healthy Body Image.* American Medical Association, 2007.

the ICD-10 specifically excludes a diagnosis for anorexia if binge eating is present.

Limitations of the criteria and proposed changes. Some research suggests that the current diagnostic criteria for eating disorders may be

TABLE 4.2

DSM-IV diagnostic criteria for anorexia nervosa

- Refusal to maintain bodyweight at or above a minimally normal weight for age and height (e.g. weight loss leading to maintenance of bodyweight less than 85% of that expected, or failure to make expected weight gain during period of growth leading to bodyweight less than 85% of that expected)

- Intense fear of gaining weight or becoming fat, even though underweight

- Disturbance in the way one's bodyweight or shape is experienced, undue influence of bodyweight or shape on self-evaluation, or denial of the seriousness of the current low bodyweight

- Amenorrhea in postmenarcheal females (i.e. the absence of at least three consecutive menstrual cycles); a woman is considered to have amenorrhea if her periods occur only following hormone (e.g. estrogen) administration

Specify type:

- *Restricting type:* during the current episode of anorexia, the person has not regularly engaged in binge-eating or purging behavior (i.e. self-induced vomiting or the misuse of laxatives, diuretics or enemas)

- *Binge-eating/purging type:* during the current episode of anorexia, the person has regularly engaged in binge-eating or purging behavior (i.e. self-induced vomiting or the misuse of laxatives, diuretics or enemas)

Adapted from the *Diagnostic and Statistical Manual of Mental Disorders,* Fourth Edition (DSM-IV). American Psychiatric Association, 2000.

too restrictive. For example, the weight criterion used in some studies has been 'at least 10% below ideal weight', which differs from the ICD-10 and DSM-IV criterion of 'at least 15% below normal or expected weight' ('less than 85% of expected weight'). The implications of the degree of weight loss, per se, are unclear, as the psychological aspects of the illness often precede weight loss, and failure to address them incipiently may result in more severe cases. Furthermore, weight-loss criteria are problematic for those patients who begin dieting at above-average weights and so are required to persist in weight-losing

TABLE 4.3
DSM-IV diagnostic criteria for bulimia nervosa

- Recurrent episodes of binge eating. An episode of binge eating is characterized by both:
  - eating, in a discrete amount of time (e.g. within any 2-hour period), an amount of food that is definitely larger (> 1000 calories) than most people would eat during a similar period of time and under similar circumstances
  - recurrent inappropriate compensatory behavior in order to prevent weight gain (e.g. self-induced vomiting, misuse of laxatives or diuretics, fasting or excessive exercise; see Classification, pages 9–10)
- The binge eating or inappropriate compensatory behaviors occur, on average, at least twice a week for 3 months
- Body shape and weight unduly influence self-evaluation and self-esteem
- The disorder must not occur only during episodes of anorexia nervosa

Specify type:

- *Purging type:* during the current episode, the patient has regularly engaged in purging behavior (i.e. self-induced vomiting or the misuse of laxatives, diuretics or enemas)
- *Non-purging type:* during the current episode, the patient has used inappropriate compensatory behaviors, such as fasting or exercising excessively, but has not regularly engaged in purging behavior (i.e. self-induced vomiting or the misuse of laxatives, diuretics or enemas)

Adapted from the *Diagnostic and Statistical Manual of Mental Disorders*, Fourth Edition (DSM-IV). American Psychiatric Association, 2000.

behaviors for longer before meeting diagnostic criteria. In either case, the use of a specific weight threshold as a diagnostic cut-off point is not based on clear scientific evidence but rather on perceived clinical significance.

The American Psychiatric Association is recommending modification of some of the diagnostic criteria for eating disorders in the coming revision of the Diagnostic and Statistical Manual of Mental Disorders (DSM-V). The suggested changes include: the removal of the amenorrhea criterion for anorexia; the listing of binge-eating disorder as a stand-alone diagnosis; and a frequency criterion of at least once a week (rather than twice a week) for binge eating and/or inappropriate compensatory behaviors in the diagnosis of bulimia or binge-eating disorder (www.DSM5.org).

Measuring weight

Accurate weight measurements are important when diagnosing an eating disorder. An adolescent patient who initially showed normal growth might stop gaining weight or might lose weight while height continues to increase. Standard procedures must be followed to record consistent reliable measurements of weight. Scales should be located in a private area, and any comments about the patient's weight should be discreet and kept to a minimum. It is important to be aware that some patients will attempt to hide their true weight by drinking extra fluids, putting weights in their pockets or even bodily orifices, or wearing lots of heavy baggy clothing and jewelry. Weighing should occur after voiding. The patient should be asked to wear a gown (when feasible) and remove all heavy objects, such as watches and jewelry.

Signs and symptoms

Although a straightforward and comprehensive clinical interview is the best way to diagnose an eating disorder, a medical examination is necessary to determine whether the symptoms observed in the patient are a result of a bio-organic or psychosocial disease. Medical causes of weight loss other than eating disorders are:
- decreased food intake because of peptic ulcer, esophageal disease, malignancy or chronic inflammatory disease
- impaired absorption because of small-bowel disease
- increased nutrient loss because of persistent diarrhea, persistent vomiting or diabetes mellitus
- excess energy demand because of hyperthyroidism, fever, malignancy, parasitic infections, cholestasis or pancreatic insufficiency.

Anorexia presents as extreme weight loss in adults, and poor or inadequate weight gain in relation to growth in children and teenagers.

Behavioral signs associated with anorexia are shown in Table 4.4.

Physical signs. The long-term effects of anorexia on the body can be alarming and severe. The typical presenting signs and symptoms are shown in Table 4.5.

TABLE 4.4

Behavioral signs of anorexia

- Rigid or obsessive behavior attached to eating (e.g. cutting food into tiny pieces, obsessive interest in what others are eating)
- Intense fear of gaining weight
- Distorted perception of body shape or weight
- Restlessness and hyperactivity
- Changes in personality; mood swings
- Wearing large baggy clothes
- Vomiting; taking laxatives
- Denial of the existence of a problem

TABLE 4.5

Physical signs and symptoms associated with starvation in anorexia nervosa

Signs	Symptoms
• Extreme weight loss in adults; poor or inadequate weight gain in children and adolescents	Fatigue
• Loss of subcutaneous tissue	
• Muscle wasting	Weakness
• Loss of bone mass	Osteoporotic fractures (in chronic cases)
• Bony protuberances	
• Acrocyanosis	Feel cold and clammy
• Lanugo (downy hair on the body)* (Figure 4.1)	

CONTINUED 37

TABLE 4.5 (CONTINUED)

• Low pulse and blood pressure	Feeling cold, lack of stamina
• Orthostatic hypotension	Dizziness
• Generalized muscle weakness	
• Peripheral neuropathy	Loss of sensation
• Dry, rough or discolored (yellow) skin	
• Scaphoid abdomen	
• Palpable stool in the left lower quadrant	Constipation and abdominal pains
• Puffy face and ankles	
• Amenorrhea (female)	Loss of interest in sex
• Absence of erections (male)	

*Sometimes hair loss on the head during recovery.

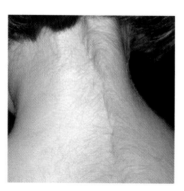

Figure 4.1 Lanugo: the soft, downy body hair that develops on the chest, back and arms of women with anorexia. © www.dermis.net

Bulimia. The typical patient with bulimia is within the normal weight range for age and height.

Behavioral signs associated with bulimia are shown in Table 4.6. Patients with bulimia often have features of depression, especially low self-esteem, and may have features of anxiety (30–70% present with depression or anxiety during their lifetime compared with a lifetime rate in the general population of 9% and 11% for mood disorders and anxiety disorders, respectively). Alcohol and substance misuse and

TABLE 4.6

Behavioral signs of bulimia (and binge eating)

- Surreptitious behavior (e.g. hiding food, spending long periods in the bathroom with vague excuses)
- Regular or excessive use of laxatives, diuretics, emetics or enemas
- Periods of fasting
- Binge eating
  - feeling out of control around food
  - eating more rapidly than usual
  - eating until feeling uncomfortably full
  - eating large amounts of food when not physically hungry
  - eating alone because of embarrassment about the quantity of food
  - self-conscious eating in front of others
  - feeling ashamed, depressed or guilty after eating
  - spontaneous regurgitation of food
- Outwardly restrictive meal patterns or overconcern with dieting and nutrition, but with little change in weight or appearance
- Dissatisfaction with body size and shape
- Excessive exercise
- Reluctance to socialize (feel helpless and alone)
- Low self-esteem, shame and guilt
- Emotional behavior and mood swings

deliberate self-harm are also common. Up to one out of two people with bulimia may report stealing.

Physical signs. Many of the physical signs and abnormalities associated with bulimia are due to recurrent vomiting (Table 4.7) and are more likely to be seen in patients with purging-type bulimia (see Classification, page 10). Medical complications include:

- gastrointestinal disorders or bleeding
- esophagitis or esophageal tears

TABLE 4.7

Physical signs and symptoms associated with bulimia

- Frequent weight changes (not necessarily weight loss)
- Tooth decay caused by loss of dental enamel due to recurrent vomiting – the loss of enamel affects the inner aspects of the front teeth in particular (see Figure 4.2)*
- Sore throat and bad breath due to excessive vomiting*
- Dehydration*
- Fatigue
- Parotid hypertrophy (swollen salivary glands making the face look rounder)
- Scars/calluses on the dorsum of the hand (Russell's sign; Figure 4.3)*
- Electrolyte disturbances*
- Esophageal or gastric tears*
- Side effects of emetics, diuretics or purgatives (e.g. dehydration, electrolyte disturbances and, in extreme cases, muscular spasms and seizures) (see Table 4.10)*
- Poor skin condition and possible hair loss
- Irregular periods
- Loss of interest in sex
- Increased risk of heart problems and problems with internal organs
- Unusual methods of adornment (e.g. tattoos, piercings)
- Direct evidence of self-harming (e.g. scars and scratches, particularly on the abdomen, thighs and arms), in case of comorbid personality disorder

*Associated with purging-type bulimia

- dental problems (Figure 4.2)
- cardiac complications (e.g. arrhythmia, tachycardia, bradycardia)
- muscle cramping due to electrolyte imbalance
- renal failure
- seizures due to hyponatremia from water overload
- hypothyroidism due to starvation.

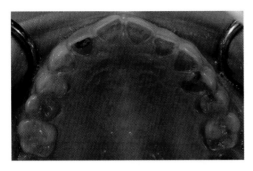

Figure 4.2 Tooth decay caused by loss of dental enamel due to recurrent vomiting. Reproduced courtesy of NYC Smile Design, New York, USA.

Cardiac complications usually arise because of nutrition- and hydration-induced electrolyte imbalance, which is pronounced in bulimia but can also occur in anorexia. These complications are generally more dangerous in patients who are underweight. Rarely, toxic substances such as diet pills, over-the-counter emetics and laxatives can induce cardiac complications.

Athletes. There is greater risk of eating disorders among competitive athletes than the general age-matched population. Females most at risk compete in aesthetic sports that encourage a slender appearance, such as gymnastics, ballet dancing, figure skating and diving, as well as in triathlon and long-distance running. Males most at risk compete in wrestling and bodybuilding. Particular signs of an eating disorder in this population include:
- excessive performance anxiety
- body dissatisfaction
- aberrant eating behaviors
- excessive training schedule/overuse injuries
- weight loss
- amenorrhea
- use of performance-enhancing drugs.

Physicians should screen adolescent and young adult athletes with questions regarding:
- weight
- possible dissatisfaction with appearance
- nutritional intake on day before screening
- amennorhea.

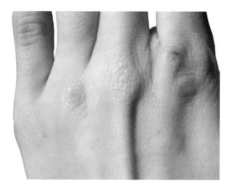

Figure 4.3 Calluses on the back of the hand (Russell's sign) caused by repeated contact of the knuckles with the incisor teeth during manual stimulation of the gag reflex to induce vomiting.

The female athlete triad. The prevalence of eating disorders in female athletes is especially high. This group often displays the 'female athlete triad':

- disordered eating
- amenorrhea
- osteoporosis.

Disordered eating does not allow sufficient nutritional intake for energy needs, resulting in hypothalamic amenorrhea. Prolonged amenorrhea can result in osteoporosis (see pages 54–5). Furthermore, female athletes often engage in periods of dietary restriction, laxative and diuretic misuse, and self-induced vomiting. Although these are common symptoms and behavioral indicators of eating disorders, most female athletes do not meet the standard criteria for anorexia or bulimia. Their bodyweight is often normal and many do not have distortion of body image. Rather, the main motivation for their behaviors is the belief that lower bodyweight will enhance athletic performance. Additionally, weight loss may be induced by comments and unrealistic demands for weight loss by coaches, particularly in aesthetic sports. Weight loss can enhance performance to some extent, but if energy expenditure is consistently below demand, this will ultimately result in loss of muscle mass and declining performance. Hence, tracking body composition

(i.e. fat versus muscle mass) is important.

Overtraining syndrome. Another presentation of disordered eating in athletes has been described as a state of exhaustion, depression and irritability in which athletes continue to train even as their athletic performance diminishes.

Diagnosis in men. Men with eating disorders are less likely than women to seek professional help, as eating disorders are commonly viewed as a 'woman's disease'. However, the number of men seeking treatment for an eating disorder may be increasing. The most common diagnosis of eating disorders among men is 'eating disorders not otherwise specified' (EDNOS). Men also exhibit higher rates of psychiatric comorbidity and psychosocial morbidity than women. Notably, men with an eating disorder – particularly bulimia or binge-eating disorder – may be more likely to have a substance-abuse problem.

Presentation can be quite different from that in women, manifesting as an emphasis on fitness and strength rather than concern with beauty and attractiveness. Anorexia is particularly difficult to diagnose in men because of the absence of the tell-tale sign of amenorrhea. When questioned effectively, men with eating disorders will report:
- nocturnal and diurnal problems with erection
- sexual dysfunction
- shrunken, and softening of, testes.

Social problems that commonly arise as a result of anorexia or bulimia include: an impaired social network, social isolation and poor social skills; reduced financial status because money is spent on purgatives and food; and impaired family relationships due to concealment and lying.

Comorbidities
Obesity. A significant yet undocumented proportion of patients with eating disorders have a history of being overweight. The excessive body dissatisfaction experienced by these patients is usually reinforced by the encouragement of weight-loss behaviors, even if these are unhealthy. Physicians should actively screen obese patients for eating disorders, and should encourage healthy eating practices, gradual

weight loss and moderation in prescribed lifestyle changes (see *Fast Facts: Obesity*).

Diabetes mellitus. Although diabetes, particularly type 2, is more prevalent in men, comorbidity of eating disorders and diabetes is seen mostly in women. Primary care physicians have an important role in identifying eating disorders in this population, as they tend to present – particularly among individuals with type 1 diabetes – as repeated medical emergencies. In addition, the complications of diabetes increase when comorbid with bulimia or EDNOS. Along with the diagnostic purging behaviors, diabetic patients may also reduce their insulin doses in attempts to control their weight. Physicians should screen all adolescents with type 1 diabetes and poor glycemic control, particularly those with rising HbA_{1c} results despite a history of good control.

Psychological conditions. The co-occurrence of eating disorders with other psychiatric syndromes has been documented in numerous studies. However, most study participants come from specialized eating-disorder clinics, so there may be an overrepresentation of more seriously compromised individuals. A large sample of mixed adults and adolescents from such a clinic found that about 63% of all patients with an eating disorder had experienced an affective disorder at some time. This comorbidity was especially high in patients with both anorexic and bulimic features.

Psychological comorbidities include:
- depression
- anxiety
- obsessive–compulsive disorder
- borderline personality disorder (more common in bulimia)
- substance misuse (see page 27).

A moderate degree of overlap between avoidant personality and anorexia has been shown in adult patients, but it remains debatable whether this applies to adolescents. Avoidant personality is described as a pervasive pattern of social inhibition. It is associated with hypersensitivity to negative evaluation, manifested as avoidance of activities that involve interpersonal contact.

Investigation

The assessment of eating disorders remains a complex clinical task, because the disorders present as a mix of disturbances in multiple domains with overlapping symptoms. A variety of diagnostic and assessment tools may be used; most are common to both anorexia and bulimia.

Structured interviews enable the reliable and valid assessment of the key behavioral features and associated psychopathology of eating disorders. The main screening tools for assessment of eating disorders are shown in Table 4.8. Other screening tools include the Rating of Anorexia and Bulimia Interview-Revised Version (RAB-R) and the Multiaxial Assessment of Eating Disorders Symptoms (MAEDS). The shortest screening instrument is certainly the SCOFF questionnaire, which is a mnemonic for the words 'Sick, Control, One (as in one stone's worth of weight, in the UK), Fat, and Food' (Table 4.9). It is a five-item tool with a score of one point given for each question that is answered affirmatively; a total of two or more points suggests an eating disorder.

Screening instruments for children include the child versions of the Eating Disorders Examination (EDE), the Eating Attitude Test (EAT), and the Eating Disorders Inventory (EDI) (see Table 4.8), as well as the Kids Eating Disorder Survey. In addition, various websites that screen for eating disorders have recently been promoted on college campuses in the USA. Data are not yet available to determine the success of these sites, but the approach is valued for its confidentiality and ease of access to younger students.

Laboratory studies may be helpful to identify the degree of electrolyte imbalance caused by frequent purging and to determine the individual's nutritional status and state of overall health. Possible biochemical abnormalities are highlighted in Table 4.10. Laboratory profiles can be followed serially to monitor fluid balance and particularly to detect hypokalemia. An electrocardiogram may be useful to detect cardiac abnormalities (see page 56).

TABLE 4.8

Screening tools for the evaluation of eating disorders

Description	Application

Eating Disorders Examination (EDE)

- 38-item semi-structured diagnostic interview
- Based on DSM-IV criteria
- Child's version available (< 14 years)
- EDE-Q self-reporting version available

- Most reliable tool for clinical evaluation
- Quantifies behaviors, symptoms and psychopathology

Eating Disorders Diagnostic Scale (EDDS)

- 22-item self-administered questionnaire

- Reliable for diagnosis of anorexia, bulimia and binge-eating disorder
- Useful for clinical and research applications

Eating Attitudes Test (EAT)

- 40-item self-administered questionnaire
- Each item rated on a 6-point scale; cut-off score for anorexia is 30
- Shorter 26-item version available (cut-off score for anorexia is 20)
- School-age child's version available

- Clinical assessment of anorexia

Eating Disorders Inventory (EDI)

- 64-item self-administered questionnaire

- Measures cognitive and behavioral factors: drive for thinness; bulimia; body dissatisfaction; ineffectiveness; perfectionism; interpersonal distrust; interoceptive awareness; maturity fears

CONTINUED

TABLE 4.8 (CONTINUED)

Structured interview for anorexic and bulimic disorders (SIAB-EX)

- 87-item structured diagnostic interview for adolescents and adults (12–65 years)
- Most items rated on a 5-point scale

- Assesses eating disorders and common associated symptoms such as depression and anxiety, specifically: body image and slimness ideal; general psychopathology; sexuality and social integration; bulimic symptoms; measures to counteract weight gain, fasting and substance abuse; atypical binges

TABLE 4.9

SCOFF questions*

Allocate 1 point for every affirmative answer: total score ≥ 2 indicates an eating disorder:

Do you make yourself **S**ick (induce vomiting) because you feel uncomfortably full?

Do you worry that you have lost **C**ontrol over how much you eat?

Have you recently lost more than **O**ne stone (14 lb [6.4 kg]) in a 3-month period?

Do you think you are too **F**at, even though others say you are too thin?

Would you say that **F**ood dominates your life?

*Positive responses to any two of these questions should prompt further investigation with a more comprehensive questionnaire (see Table 4.8). Adapted from Morgan JF, Reid F, Lacey JH. The SCOFF questionnaire: assessment of a new screening tool for eating disorders. *BMJ* 1999;319:1467–8.

Differential diagnosis

Anorexia. After ensuring that the patient's weight loss is not due to a medical condition, the major considerations are:

- major depression accompanied by weight loss from appetite suppression and low mood

TABLE 4.10

Biochemical abnormalities associated with eating disorders

- Mild anemia
- Low erythrocyte sedimentation rate
- Hypokalemia*
- Hypochloremia*
- Hyponatremia*
- Metabolic alkalosis[†]
- Metabolic acidosis[‡]
- Low triiodothyronine (T3) level
- Occasionally low thyroxine (T4) level
- Elevated amylase from vomiting

*Caused by frequent purging.
[†]Caused by loss of stomach acid due to vomiting.
[‡]Caused by frequent self-induced diarrhea.

- psychotic disorder involving paranoid or delusional beliefs regarding eating or weight
- obsessive–compulsive disorder involving rituals about food and weight that are undesired or in conflict with the patient's self-perception.

Careful interview of the patient, family members and other clinicians may be required to clarify the diagnosis.

Bulimia. The most common differential diagnoses of bulimia are:
- binge-eating disorder
- anorexia nervosa
- gastrointestinal disorders.

Binge-eating disorder is characterized by bingeing without compensatory behaviors of either purging or non-purging type. There is no body distortion or overconcern with body image.

Anorexia may also involve bingeing and purging, but not as consistently as bulimia. Patients with anorexia must be at least 15% below the expected bodyweight, whereas there is often weight fluctuation and no recognizable weight loss in patients with bulimia.

Key points – diagnosis

- Both DSM-IV and ICD-10 provide specific criteria for the diagnosis of bulimia and anorexia.
- Structured interviews allow the reliable and valid assessment of the key behavioral features and associated psychopathology of eating disorders.
- Patients with eating disorders are likely to present with profound weight loss or weight fluctuations, malnutrition and a number of medical complications associated with recurrent vomiting, as well as social problems.
- Comorbid psychological problems include depression, anxiety and obsessive behavior, and substance misuse in patients with bulimia.
- Laboratory tests may help to identify the degree of electrolyte imbalance caused by frequent purging and to determine overall nutritional status and need for hospitalization.

Key references

American Psychiatric Association. *Practice Guidelines for the Treatment of Psychiatric Disorders, Compendium 2006; Eating Disorders*, 3rd edn. Washington, DC: American Psychiatric Association, 2006.

Cooper Z, Fairburn CG. The Eating Disorder Examination: a semi-structured interview for the assessment of the specific psychopathology of eating disorders. *Int J Eat Dis* 1987;6:1–8.

Corcos M, Nezelof S, Speranza M et al. Psychoactive substance consumption in eating disorders. *Eat Behav* 2001;2:27–38.

Fichter MM, Quadflieg N. The structured interview for anorexic and bulimic disorders for DSM-IV and ICD-10 (SIAB-EX): reliability and validity. *Eur Psychiatry* 2001;16: 38–48.

Garner DM, Garfinkel PE. The Eating Attitudes Test: an index of the symptoms of anorexia nervosa. *Psychol Med* 1979;9:273–9.

Garner DM, Olmstead MP. *Manual for Eating Disorder Inventory (EDI)*. Odessa: Psychological Assessment Resource, 1984.

Golden, NH. Eating disorders in adolescence and their sequelae. *Best Pract Res Clin Obstet Gynaecol* 2003:17: 57–73.

Grant BF, Stinson FS, Dawson DA et al. Prevalence and co-occurrence of substance use disorders and independent mood and anxiety disorders. Results from the National Epidemiologic Survey on Alcohol and Related Conditions. *Arch Gen Psychiatry* 2004;61:807–16.

Haslam D, Wittert G. *Fast Facts: Obesity*. Oxford: Health Press, 2009.

Luck AJ, Morgan JF, Reid F et al. The SCOFF questionnaire and clinical interview for eating disorders in general practice: comparative study. *BMJ* 2002;325:755–6.

Sigman, GS. Eating disorders in children and adolescents. *Pediatr Clin N Am* 2003:50:1139–77.

WHO. *International Statistical Classification of Behavioral Disorders*, 10th edn. Geneva: World Health Organization, 1992.

The multidisciplinary team

Treatment of eating disorders requires a multidisciplinary team of professionals to provide the appropriate care for the patient. This team usually consists of a primary medical physician, a psychotherapist and/or psychiatrist and a dietitian. It is the responsibility of every team member to inform each other, as well as appropriate family members, of the patient's state. Together, the team decides what type of treatment is necessary along the continuum of care:

- outpatient therapy
- partial hospitalization
- inpatient care
- residential care.

The interventions used in treatment need to be developmentally appropriate. As this is a complex multifactorial group of disorders, caregivers must anticipate long-term care, as treatment may require months or even years.

The primary care physician, throughout treatment, has several important functions:

- to diagnose and treat any chronic and/or acute symptoms and complications
- to monitor the patient's physiological status, including shifts in weight, blood pressure, pulse and other cardiovascular parameters
- to continually reappraise the patient's physical state in order to confront any denial
- to inform other members of the treatment team and appropriate family members of the patient's physical state.

The psychiatrist/psychotherapist also plays an important role throughout treatment. In one treatment model, the psychiatrist or psychotherapist solely manages the psychological needs of the patient; in another model, the psychiatrist manages both the general medical and psychological needs, with specialized assistance from a psychotherapist. In either model, the psychiatrist or psychotherapist has the following responsibilities:

- to assess eating-disorder symptoms and behaviors
- to monitor the patient's psychological status, including behavior shifts, cognitions, and emotions
- to provide individual, family or group psychotherapy.

The dietitian oversees the nutritional counseling of the patient, providing several important functions:

- to ensure adequate nutrient intake
- to improve dietary variety
- to establish structured normalized eating patterns to help address detrimental attitudes towards food and eating
- to provide education regarding healthy nutrition and eating patterns.

Treatment goals

The ultimate goal of treatment is both psychological and physical health. It is important to emphasize these definitions of recovery as opposed to defining recovery simply as weight gain or a temporary change in behavior.

Psychological health involves the development of normal eating behaviors, without restricting or purging, and the elimination of obsessions with body image, bodyweight and food. The psychological aspects of treatment can be divided into three levels:

- interrupting pathological food-related behaviors
- treating pathological coping and precipitating factors
- treating perpetuating factors.

Physical health is attained when weight and menses have been restored in anorexia. In bulimia, the goal is complete discontinuation of any purging behaviors. The medical aspect of treatment involves monitoring for common complications such as:

- gastrointestinal symptoms
- cardiac symptoms

- oligomenorrhea or amenorrhea
- reductions in bone density
- side effects of psychopharmacological agents.

  Acute problems of eating disorders include:
- fluid, electrolyte and acid-base abnormalities
- cardiac rhythm disturbances
- edema
- gastrointestinal symptoms such as delayed gastric emptying, constipation, irritable colon symptoms and esophageal disease (e.g. esophagitis, ruptures).

  Chronic problems include:
- growth retardation
- pubertal arrest
- amenorrhea
- oligomenorrhea
- impaired acquisition of peak bone mass
- cerebral atrophy
- chronic renal tubular disease.

There are also potentially irreversible problems associated with chronic eating disorders (Table 5.1). Sudden death is also possible.

TABLE 5.1

Potentially irreversible consequences of eating disorders

- Growth retardation in the presence of normal menses
- Abnormal pubertal development
- Bone loss and impaired acquisition of peak bone mass
- Abnormalities of reproductive capacity
- Cerebral atrophy, chronic renal tubular disease
- Ventricular arrhythmia (hypokalemia, long QT interval and torsades de pointes)
- Esophageal or gastric rupture
- Re-feeding hypophosphatemia
- Congestive heart failure

Management of complications

Amenorrhea is a key feature of anorexia in particular. It is a consequence of a disturbance in the regulation of hypothalamic secretion of gonadotrophin-releasing hormone. This results in low levels of luteinizing hormone (LH), follicle-stimulating hormone and estradiol, a prepubertal pattern of LH pulsatile secretion, and a regression of uterus and ovary size. Prolonged amenorrhea can lead to osteopenia, which is a precursor to osteoporosis (see below).

Weight gain is important for the restoration of menses; 86% of patients who achieve 90% of their ideal bodyweight resume menses within 6 months.

Low bone density

Osteopenia is the most serious, potentially irreversible complication of the low estrogen levels caused by prolonged amenorrhea. Nutritional factors also play an important role, as indicated by the more serious cases of osteopenia in anorexia compared with hypothalamic amenorrhea. In osteopenia, the level of markers of bone formation decrease and those of bone resorption increase. Osteopenia is defined by a bone mineral density (BMD) of 1.0–2.5 standard deviations (SDs) below the young adult reference mean. BMD is most commonly measured by means of dual-energy X-ray absorptiometry (DEXA). For children and adolescents, readings should be compared with the reference ranges for healthy young adults (T-scores) and age-matched children and adolescents (Z-scores) (Figure 5.1).

During adolescence, individuals develop 60% of peak bone mass; very little bone mass is accumulated from 2 years after menarche. Again, weight gain is crucial as an increase in BMD relies primarily on bodyweight. Patients who achieve more than 85% of their ideal bodyweight show significant improvement in spinal bone mass.

Osteoporosis is a clinical syndrome resulting from decreased bone mass and disruption of the normal bone microarchitecture (see *Fast Facts: Osteoporosis*). It is defined by a BMD greater than 2.5 SDs below the mean for young adult women (a T-score of –1 to –2.5). Hormone replacement therapy has not been shown to be effective at

increasing bone mass in the treatment of eating disorders. Weight gain

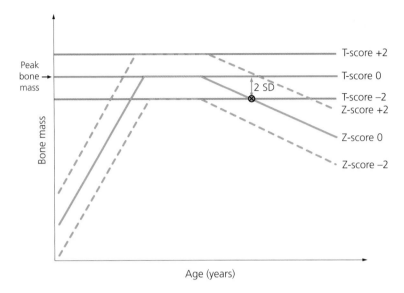

Figure 5.1 The derivation of T- and Z-scores. The point marked by the cross demonstrates a bone mass value lying two standard deviations (SDs) below the mean reference value for premenopausal women (peak bone mass) and therefore illustrates a T-score of –2. The dotted lines indicate Z-scores of +2 and –2.

is vital to improving bone mass. Calcium supplements (minimum 1000 mg/day), vitamin D (400 IU/day) and moderate weight-bearing exercise are also commonly prescribed.

Other promising treatments are being investigated, such as oral dehydroepiandrosterone (DHEA), human insulin-like growth factor 1 (rhIGF-I), and zoledronic acid (zoledronate). Varying doses of DHEA over a 3-month period showed some improvement in bone turnover and osteocalcin levels, but no significant improvements in BMD and body composition.

Gastrointestinal symptoms. The following gastrointestinal symptoms are common in patients with eating disorders, particularly during the weight-restoration phase:
- abdominal pain
- bloating

- constipation
- delayed gastric emptying
- irritable bowel syndrome (IBS).

As fear of eating and weight gain is characteristic of these patients, it may be difficult to distinguish between psychological distress and actual physical discomfort. Aggressive treatment is not necessary because these symptoms are adaptive and tend to resolve as normal eating patterns are established. However, the following medications can be prescribed to alleviate gastrointestinal symptoms:

- anticholinergic agents or selective serotonin-reuptake inhibitors (SSRIs) for IBS
- peristaltic agents such as metoclopramide for postprandial bloating
- non-purging agents with fiber, mineral oil or polyethylene glycol for constipation.

Referral to a specialist is recommended for esophageal complications.

Cardiac symptoms. An electrocardiogram may reveal:

- bradycardia
- low-voltage complexes
- non-specific ST-segment depression
- T-wave changes
- a prolonged QTc interval.

Sinus bradycardia with rates lower than 30 beats per minute is a characteristic complication of malnutrition. This symptom is adaptive and will resolve with weight gain. If there is no junctional escape or other arrhythmia then the standard treatment for anorexia is sufficient. If the QTc interval is prolonged and dispersed, however, there is a risk of ventricular arrhythmia and sudden death. Inpatient admission may be needed for:

- cardiac monitoring
- rapid nutritional repletion
- evaluation of electrolyte abnormalities.

Side effects of psychopharmacological agents include:

- rapid weight loss and gain (with SSRIs and atypical antipsychotics)
- carbohydrate cravings

- nausea
- sleep disturbance – hypersomnia and hyposomnia
- night sweats (with SSRIs)
- agitation
- increased risk for suicide ideation
- induction of bulimia
- menstrual irregularity/amenorrhea.

Follow-up

Ongoing monitoring is driven by:

- acuity of the weight loss
- extent of malnutrition
- frequency and acuity of vomiting and compensatory behaviors
- drug and dietary control of medication abuse.

Initially, the acuity of weight loss dictates the frequency of follow-up, so some patients may require multiple weekly check-ups in an effort to

---

Key points – general management principles

- The treatment of eating disorders requires a multidisciplinary team of healthcare professionals, involving the primary care physician, psychiatrist and nutritionist.
- The ultimate goal of treatment is both psychological and physical health.
- Psychological health comprises: healthy eating behaviors with no restricting or purging; the elimination of obsessions regarding body image, bodyweight and food; normal adaptive functioning in school/work and interpersonal relationships; and coping with normative stressors.
- Physical health is measured by the restoration of ideal bodyweight and return of menses.
- There are many complications, acute and chronic, associated with eating disorders that require ongoing management.
- Weight gain is crucial in order to restore menses and increase bone density.

avoid hospitalization. In the weight-restoration phase patients should be seen weekly. As patients achieve weight gain beyond the 85% ideal, and approaching 100%, they can be seen less frequently and monthly visits may suffice. When patients are asymptomatic and weight is restored, follow-up visits can be as infrequent as once or twice a year for 4 years after onset, as this is the period in which patients are generally considered vulnerable to relapse.

The information to be obtained at each visit is shown in Table 5.2.

TABLE 5.2

Information to obtain at each follow-up visit

- Daily energy intake
- Menstrual status
- Frequency of vomiting per week or day
- Height
- Weight (in gown and after voiding)
- Body mass index
- Orthostatic vital signs and body temperature (to detect hypothermia; see Table 6.1)
- Specific gravity and pH of urine
- Electrolytes, if vomiting or pronounced weight gain or loss
- Serum amylase, if reported or suspected vomiting (see page 45)
- Ad hoc laboratory tests and electrocardiogram to follow up on cardiac status, malnutrition and long-term effects of amenorrhea (depending on symptoms)

Key references

American Psychiatric Association. *Practice Guidelines for the Treatment of Psychiatric Disorders, Compendium 2006; Eating Disorders*, 3rd edn. Washington, DC: American Psychiatric Association, 2006.

Compston J, Rosen C. *Fast Facts: Osteoporosis*, 5th edn. Oxford: Health Press, 2009.

Golden NH. Osteopenia and osteoporosis in anorexia nervosa. *Adolesc Med* 2003;14:97–108.

Golden NH. Eating disorders in adolescence: what is the role of hormone replacement therapy? *Curr Opin Obstet Gynecol* 2007;19:434–39.

Golden NH, Iglesias EA, Jacobson MS et al. Alendronate for the treatment of osteopenia in anorexia nervosa: a randomized, double-blind, placebo-controlled trial. *J Clin Endocrinol Metab* 2005;90:3179–85.

Golden NH, Lanzkowsky L, Schebendach J et al. The effect of estrogen-progestin treatment on bone mineral density in anorexia nervosa. *J Ped Adolesc Gynecol* 2002;15: 135–43.

Grinspoon S, Thomas L, Miller K et al. Effects of recombinant human IGF-I and oral contraceptive administration on bone density in anorexia nervosa. *J Clin Endocrinol Metab* 2002;87:2883–91.

Klibanski A, Biller BM, Schoenfeld DA et al. The effects of estrogen administration on trabecular bone loss in young women with anorexia nervosa. *J Clin Endocrinol Metab* 1995;80:898–904.

Sigman GS. Eating disorders in children and adolescents. *Pediatr Clin N Am* 2003:50:1139–1177.

Much of the treatment of anorexia is based on limited clinical evidence and is likely to remain so given the difficulty of carrying out clinical trials on this relatively rare disorder.

Treatment approach

Rapid identification of the condition and early intervention is of paramount importance given the definitive evidence that patients with a duration of illness of less than 1–2 years, particularly adolescents and those with reasonably functional families, have a higher chance of recovery.

The evidence indicates that individual, familial, nutritional, medical and psychological aspects of anorexia should all be addressed using a comprehensive and multidisciplinary approach. Guidelines for the psychiatric and medical treatment of anorexia have been published, for example by the American Psychiatric Association, the UK National Institute for Health and Clinical Excellence (NICE), the American Academy of Pediatrics, and the Society for Adolescent Health and Medicine.

The primary goals of treatment for anorexia are to:
- restore patients to a healthy weight associated with:
  - return of menses and normal ovulation (in females)
  - normal sex drive and hormone levels (in males)
  - normal physical and sexual growth and development (in children and adolescents)
- help patients learn, regain and maintain healthy eating patterns
- address other psychological issues related to the primary diagnosis of anorexia
- restore the parental role to create a functioning parenting unit (for children and adolescents).

Hospitalization

Table 6.1 shows the indications for hospitalization of adolescents with anorexia. In the USA, under the influence of managed care and in the absence of a national health plan, the role of hospitalization for anorexia has changed dramatically over the past 10 years. In some EU countries

TABLE 6.1

Indications for hospitalization in adolescents with anorexia

- Severe malnutrition ($\leq$ 85% average bodyweight for age, height and sex)
- Dehydration
- Serious electrolyte or metabolic abnormalities (e.g. hypokalemia, hyponatremia, hypophosphatemia)
- Cardiac dysrhythmia
- Physiological instability
  - severe bradycardia (daytime HR < 50 beats/min; night-time HR < 45 beats/min)
  - hypotension (< 80/50 mmHg)
  - hypothermia (body temperature < 35.6°C)
  - orthostatic changes in pulse (> 20 beats/min) or blood pressure (> 10 mmHg)
- Arrested growth and development
- Rapid and persistent decline in oral intake or weight despite intensive outpatient treatment
- Acute food refusal
- Uncontrollable bingeing and/or purging
- Acute medical complications of malnutrition (e.g. syncope, seizures, cardiac failure, pancreatitis)
- Acute psychiatric emergency (e.g. suicidal ideation, acute psychosis)
- Comorbid condition that interferes with treatment (e.g. severe depression, obsessive–compulsive disorder, severe family dysfunction)

HR, heart rate.
Adapted from Eating disorders in adolescents: position paper of the Society for Adolescent Medicine. *J Adolesc Health* 2003;33:496–503.
www.adolescenthealth.org/PositionPaper_Eating_Disorders_in_Adolescents.pdf

and Australia, where national health plans are in operation, hospitalization has remained a major tool for weight rehabilitation and initial treatment. The average length of hospital stay in the USA is about 1–2 weeks, with inpatient treatment limited to brief acute weight restoration and nutritional rehabilitation (Table 6.2). Conversely, in other industrialized nations, it is not uncommon for patients to spend several weeks or even months in hospital in the initial treatment phase.

Unfortunately, a low discharge weight may create an unnecessary risk for relapse and poor prognosis. Studies report that up to 40% of hospitalized patients with anorexia are readmitted at least once. The length of stay becomes longer with each successive hospitalization. Inpatient treatment studies of young adults suggest a continued role for hospitalization for severe cases. The Society of Adolescent Medicine's

TABLE 6.2

Key elements of nutritional rehabilitation

- Controlled weight gain: 2–3 lb/week (0.9–1.4 kg) for inpatients (0.5–1 lb/week [0.2–0.5 kg] for outpatients)
- Intake levels starting at 30–40 kcal/kg/day in divided meals
- Detection of circulatory overload, re-feeding edema and bloating by daily assessment of:
  - morning weight
  - vital signs
  - fluid intake
  - urine output
- Monitoring of serum electrolyte levels
- Electrocardiogram (if required)
- Stool softeners (not laxatives) to treat constipation
- Vitamin and mineral supplements
- Positive reinforcers (praise)
- Negative reinforcers (restrictions on exercise and purging)
- Close supervision
- Restricted access to bathrooms (for about 2 hours after meals)

publication of medical treatment guidelines suggests a consistent pattern of acute hospitalization for patients with anorexia (see Table 6.1).

Non-pharmacological treatment

Despite the lack of solid data backing up the efficacy of non-pharmacological treatment, clinicians and clinical researchers agree that psychotherapeutic intervention is the mainstay of treatment for anorexia across all age groups. Because of the high cost of inpatient treatment and its disruptive effect on normal adolescent life, various outpatient approaches to individual, family and group therapy have been employed in the treatment of anorexia. The literature on the comparative efficacy of various psychological approaches in anorexia is very limited (three controlled trials) and does not demonstrate any significant difference between the therapies considered:

- psychodynamic therapy
- cognitive–behavior therapy (CBT)
- family therapy or supportive therapy.

Most clinicians base their interventions for adolescent patients on one of three models: individual psychodynamic therapy, family therapy and family-based treatment. The use of cognitive behavioral techniques is an integral part of most multimodal treatment programs for anorexia, whether on an outpatient or inpatient basis. However, rigorous efficacy treatment studies of intensive full-time or day treatment programs are few, especially in adolescents.

Psychotherapy has been shown to be ineffective during the acute re-feeding stage of treatment, although a therapeutic alliance is helpful in increasing patient motivation. The therapeutic alliance has been broadly defined as the affective and collaborative bond between patient and therapist in which the patient feels positive about the therapist, perceives there to be a shared valuation of treatment tasks, and considers the intervention activities to be helpful. Psychotherapy is believed to be more helpful after weight restoration, although further formal study is needed.

Psychodynamic therapy aims to increase the patient's self-awareness so that they can understand how past or present dysfunctional relationships   63 or experiences have manifested as the current eating disorder. This form of therapy takes a global approach, not only addressing the dysfunctional behavior but the restoration of overall functioning. Typical topics addressed are relationships to significant others (especially parents), female role expectations and conflicts regarding pubertal development and adult demands. By focusing on and addressing these issues the patient is able to change the disordered eating behavior and resume normal development. The emphasis on symptom reduction and simultaneous expectation of normalization of functioning characterizes psychodynamic treatment of anorexia. In a recent review of meta-analyses of this form of treatment, the author concluded that "the available evidence indicates that effect sizes for psychodynamic therapies are as large as those reported for other treatments that have been actively promoted as "empirically supported" and "evidence based" (e.g. CBT and anti-anxiolytics/antidepressants).

Although there are no head-to-head controlled clinical trials in the psychotherapy of eating disorders, in the light of surprising and encouraging findings, we suggest future studies be tracked very closely.

Cognitive–behavior therapy is less firmly established in the treatment of anorexia than of bulimia. There are no studies for the exact phasing of treatment, but the overall goal mirrors that of bulimia treatment (see Chapter 7). The patient is asked to self-monitor nutritional intake, as well as behaviors and attitudes towards eating, weight and shape to track and expose dysfunctional beliefs and attitudes. Cognitive restructuring of dysfunctional thoughts is accomplished through education about healthy eating behaviors and adaptive coping behaviors.

Minimal research exists on the effectiveness of CBT for anorexic patients, largely because of the difficulties associated with conducting research in this patient population. A small controlled trial evaluating the efficacy of CBT as a post-hospitalization treatment for anorexia in adults found reduced relapse rates and improved outcomes.

In randomized controlled trials in patients with anorexia, CBT was not found to be superior to other types of treatment such as psychoanalytic psychotherapy, cognitive–analytic therapy, family therapy for 1 year and low-contact routine treatment. However, adherence to treatment was better with CBT, suggesting that this technique may be more acceptable to patients than other psychological treatments.

Family therapy. Because family attitudes can have a major role in the development of eating disorders (see page 21), the familial relationships of patients with early-onset anorexia should be examined. Family therapy is best started after a hospitalized patient has gained weight, but before discharge; it should be continued after the patient has left hospital. Parents can unintentionally collaborate in their child's illness; for example, they may identify with the goal of thinness and not perceive that their child is unhealthily underweight. In such cases, they need to understand the danger of the disorder and how to avoid encouraging unhealthy behavior.

At present, the most evidence-based approach to anorexia treatment, particularly in adolescents, is family therapy. In one of the most successful treatment model interventions, the Maudsley family therapy method, developed at the Maudsley Hospital in London, UK, the parents are encouraged to take charge of the patient's eating until weight is restored and normal eating resumed. This is in sharp contrast to traditional approaches in which dieting and weight restoration is managed by the 'experts'. This model seems to have short- and long-term benefits in those able to participate. However, many families do not agree to participate and thus need to be managed according to their particular needs.

Published studies have considered family interventions during hospitalization and during outpatient treatments. Various family therapies (e.g. psychodynamic, cognitive, systemic, psychoeducative) have been shown to have a positive effect on the adolescent's weight. Family treatment appears to produce good results at the start of the disorder in young adolescents, but it does not produce savings in hospitalization in some severe life-threatening forms of the disease. In addition, taking the family dynamic into consideration in the treatment plan appears to have a specific effect on overall improvement in addition to weight gain.

One systematic review states that where serious discord exists within the family it may be preferable to consider individual psychotherapy for the anorexic patient, with accompanying support, information and assistance for the parents. Depending on the case, direct face-to-face meetings between the patient and the parents can have a positive influence on the relationship or can heighten conflict. The therapist's clinical judgment on an individual case-by-case basis is essential.

Other psychological approaches such as motivational enhancement therapy (MET) and experiential non-verbal therapies are promising. Non-specific factors inherent in the psychotherapeutic process are important for patients with an illness such as anorexia: warmth and genuineness, understanding and acceptance, and openness and honesty are all essential components that clinicians must provide to help remove the sense of isolation and aloneness patients feel.

Psychopharmacological treatment

As for the psychotherapies, which are still considered the mainstay of anorexia treatment, the evidence base and, moreover, consensus on the most effective psychopharmacological treatments of anorexia are limited, in contrast to the treatment of bulimia. Furthermore, anorexic patients often refuse this type of intervention out of concern that they would gain too much weight too quickly.

Generally, it is recommended to wait until weight is restored before administering drug treatments because eating-disorder symptoms and associated psychopathological features (such as anxiety and depression) may remit with weight gain. Furthermore, the side effects of medications may complicate the effects of malnutrition and the re-feeding process unnecessarily. However, in severe cases where the patient is unable to gain significant weight or presents with severe comorbid psychopathology, medications can be administered before complete weight restoration to address:

- anxiety about re-feeding
- increasing depression and discouragement due to lack of progress
- obsessional features activated by the re-feeding
- bulimic behavior
- in rare cases, transient psychotic states induced by severe malnutrition.

Antipsychotics. Patients with anorexia have long been treated with traditional antipsychotic medication because their obsession regarding weight and body shape seemed to resemble delusions. More recently, the atypical antipsychotics have been used for their anti-anxiety effect, as well as their higher ratio of serotonin-to-dopamine blockade, associated with a much more favorable side-effect profile, which often includes impressive weight gain. As yet, however, there have been only three small controlled studies supporting the efficacy of an atypical antipsychotic (olanzapine) in adults with anorexia, and only case reports and small series for adolescents with the disorder.

It is best to consider the second-generation antipsychotics as treatments of last resort for extremely malnourished, severely ill patients with severe resistance to weight gain and severe obsessional thinking, often bordering on psychotic delusions and anxieties. The main problem is that the dopaminergic blockade produced by these medications often induces hyperphagia, leading to bulimic episodes that terrify the patient. In addition, the risk of cardiac complications such as QTc prolongation, tardive dyskinesia and other movement disorders, neuroleptic malignant syndrome and hyperprolactinemia may make the safe use of drugs difficult in this population. Treatment should be started under extremely close supervision, ideally in a hospital setting, and discontinued once weight rehabilitation has achieved some sustained momentum.

Olanzapine and risperidone are two potent atypical antipsychotics that have been reported to have a positive effect on weight gain and to induce symptomatic improvement of anxiety/agitation, obsessive thoughts, paranoid ideation and compulsive hyperenergetic activity. Olanzapine can be given at 5–12.5 mg/day and is the only medication which has demonstrated an adjunctive effect for inpatient treatment of underweight women with anorexia in controlled studies; risperidone has been used at doses of 0.5–1.5 mg/day. Reported adverse reactions have been limited to initial sedation. Both of these drugs are known to produce rapid and large weight gain, which very quickly becomes apparent to the patient and rapidly leads to non-adherence to the regimen. A reasonable strategy to circumvent these problems in severe cases is to start at very low doses (5 mg olanzapine, 0.5 mg risperidone) that remain effective in reducing anxiety about re-feeding.

Quetiapine and aripiprazole are two newer agents that may have fewer side effects with preserved efficacy. Quetiapine has been given at 50–800 mg/day and aripiprazole at 30 mg/day, although there is no scientific evidence for efficacy in this indication.

Other antipsychotics, atypical and typical, are either untested or no more effective than placebo in controlled trials.

Antidepressants target the extremely common symptoms of depression, anxiety or obsessive–compulsive symptoms. Although theoretically this type of medication should be useful in patients with anorexia, the results from controlled studies have been disappointing. Many of these drugs are slow to work (as a rule, a matter of weeks) and many can disinhibit eating and lead to weight gain, a side effect dreaded by this patient population. Some patients report considerable and uncontrollable carbohydrate hunger. Night sweats, sedation and somnolence are all bothersome side effects. It is best to use the newer selective serotonin-reuptake inhibitors (SSRIs) and selective norepinephrine (noradrenaline)-reuptake inhibitors (SNRIs), because older tricyclic compounds have pronounced anticholinergic and cardiovascular side effects that complicate the re-feeding process. These compounds downregulate the anxiety system and treat mood problems that persist after weight rehabilitation. However, the lack of persuasive evidence of efficacy in patients with anorexia even after weight restoration raises the important question as to whether these compounds can perform well in a recently malnourished person.

Clinicians have increasingly turned to SSRIs over the past two decades. However, the research on treatment of anorexia with SSRIs has not been particularly promising. Additional research is needed to establish the possible efficacy of SSRIs in preventing relapse in weight-restored individuals with anorexia. Two compounds have been studied, fluoxetine and citalopram, with very mixed results.

Fluoxetine. There is still no agreement regarding the efficacy of fluoxetine in anorexic patients. Studies have shown no significant benefits when prescribed during the weight restoration phase, but a study during the first year of weight maintenance after successful inpatient treatment demonstrated that fluoxetine, up to 60 mg/day, prevented relapse in women with anorexia. Another study showed no benefit following weight restoration, and fluoxetine was not found to be superior to placebo for inpatients with anorexia who were also receiving behavioral therapy.

Citalopram. During the weight restoration phase this SSRI may decrease the associated symptoms of depression and anxiety but it has not been shown to increase the rate of weight gain. One study demonstrated an alarming drop in bodyweight (mean 5.4 kg) and an overall response worse than placebo. If using this agent, clinicians should monitor the patient's weight closely.

Tricyclic antidepressants such as amitriptyline and clomipramine should not be used in patients with anorexia. Randomized controlled trials have produced negative results. Underweight patients are particularly prone to the side effects of tricyclic antidepressants. There is a potential for arrhythmia at low bodyweight, plus a risk of lethal overdose and concern surrounding sudden death in young people. Additionally, prescription of tricyclic antidepressants should be avoided for suicidal patients and patients with cardiovascular concerns.

Mood-stabilizing medications such as lithium have not been effective in patients with anorexia.

Other pharmacological treatments
Other medications have been tried for the treatment of anorexia but have not demonstrated efficacy in published trials.

Prokinetic agents (medications that improve gastric emptying), i.e. metoclopramide, bethanechol and domperidone, have been suggested as possible adjuvants to help patients with anorexia to eat; however, some of these drugs have a depressant effect on the central nervous system and none has been studied with a controlled design.

Opioid antagonists. Anorexic patients often characterize their behavior as addictive, and there are similarities between eating disorders and substance-use disorders. Consequently, the opioid antagonists such as naltrexone have been considered a treatment option for anorexia. There was a lot of excitement when this drug appeared 15 years ago; however, there is no evidence of efficacy of naltrexone or related compounds in this population and as such they are not administered.

Cyproheptadine, a serotonin and histamine antagonist that can produce weight gain in the treatment of children with asthma, has been tested for women with anorexia in two controlled studies. Weight gain did not differ between patients receiving the active drug and those on placebo, and other investigators have not been able to replicate the one favorable study in the literature.

Zinc supplementation. Individuals with zinc deficiency exhibit symptoms similar to those of patients with anorexia, i.e. weight loss, depression, changes in appetite and taste, and amenorrhea. Given the nutritional deprivation in anorexic patients and therefore the likelihood of zinc deficiency there was a potential role for zinc supplementation. Three controlled studies have been conducted in children and adolescents, but the results have been mixed and the role of zinc deficiency in the pathogenesis of anorexia remains controversial.

Optimizing treatment

Anorexia should not be thought of as a prime disorder for psychopharmacological interventions, especially in isolation. Medications, at the present time, have a predominantly adjunctive role, and many of their side effects may complicate the nutritional rehabilitation of the patient. Certainly no medication is curative in this indication.

The measured and empathic re-feeding process, facilitated by psychotherapeutic interventions with the family and the patient, is the best combination leading to recovery. Nutritional rehabilitation is the backbone on which recovery becomes possible. Psychotherapy helps build a treatment alliance, with both the patient and the parents, to maximize compliance with prescribed weight gain. Medications are used with careful supervision to target specific complications that arise during this process in patients' dire distress, and facilitate the return of an orderly treatment progression.

Key points – treatment of anorexia

- Up to 40% of patients with anorexia are readmitted to the hospital at least once for weight restoration and nutritional rehabilitation; the length of stay becomes longer with each successive hospitalization.
- Cognitive–behavior therapy and other psychotherapeutic techniques are an integral part of most multimodal treatment programs for anorexia, for both outpatients and inpatients.
- Patients with anorexia can be treated with antipsychotic medication in dire situations and in crises, as these medications become effective relatively quickly. Appropriate targets are the patient's obsession regarding weight and body shape (which often resemble a delusion), extreme anxiety regarding re-feeding, and psychotic states.
- Some second-generation atypical antipsychotics such as olanzapine, risperidone, quetiapine and aripiprazole have a more favorable side-effect profile than the traditional antipsychotics, including a higher ratio of serotonin-to-dopamine blockade and weight gain.
- Tricyclic antidepressants are not recommended for the treatment of patients with anorexia because of the potential for arrhythmia at low bodyweight, a risk of lethal overdose and concern surrounding sudden death in young people.
- Selective serotonin-reuptake inhibitors (SSRIs) can target anxiety and depression if efficacy is not of immediate concern. They have a more manageable side-effect profile than the atypical antipsychotics, but treatment should be monitored carefully for suicidality, weight gain or loss, emotional activation and agitation.
- Further research is needed to establish the efficacy of SSRIs in preventing relapse in weight-restored individuals.

Key references

American Psychiatric Association. *Practice Guidelines for the Treatment of Psychiatric Disorders, Compendium 2006; Eating Disorders*, 3rd edn. Washington, DC: American Psychiatric Association, 2006.

Attia E, Haiman C, Walsh BT, Flater SR. Does fluoxetine augment the inpatient treatment of anorexia nervosa? *Am J Psychiatry* 1998; 155:548–51.

Bissada H, Tasca G, Barber AM, Bradwejn J. Olanzapine in the treatment of low body weight and obsessive thinking in women with anorexia nervosa: A randomized, double-blind, placebo-controlled trial. *Am J Psychiatry* 2008:165:1281–8.

Dare C, Eisler I, Russell G et al. Psychological therapies for adults with anorexia nervosa: randomised controlled trial of out-patient treatments. *Br J Psychiatry* 2001;178:216–21.

Flament MF, Bissada H, Spettigue W. Evidence-based pharmacotherapy of eating disorders. *Int J Neuropsychopharmacol* 2011. Epub ahead of print (doi: 10.1017/S1461145711000381).

Kachele H, Kordy H, Richard M et al. Therapy amount and outcome of inpatient psychodynamic treatment of eating disorders in Germany: data from a multicenter study. *Psychother Res* 2001;11: 239–57.

Kaplan AS. Psychological treatments for anorexia nervosa: a review of published studies and promising new directions. *Can J Psychiatry* 2002;47: 235–42.

Kaye WH, Nagata T, Weltzin TE et al. Double-blind placebo-controlled administration of fluoxetine in restricting and restricting-purging-type anorexia nervosa. *Biol Psychiatry* 2001;49:644–52.

Le Grange D, Lock J. The dearth of psychological treatment studies for anorexia nervosa. *Int J Eat Disorders* 2005:37:79–81.

Lock J, Le Grange D, Agras WS et al. Randomized clinical trial comparing family-based treatment with adolescent-focused individual therapy for adolescents with anorexia nervosa. *Arch Gen Psychiatry* 2010;67:1025–32.

Mitchell JE, de Zwaan M, Roerig JL. Drug therapy for patients with eating disorders. *Curr Drug Targets CNS Neurol Disord* 2003;2:17–19.

National Collaborating Centre for Mental Health. *Eating Disorders. Core interventions in the treatment and management of anorexia nervosa, bulimia nervosa, and related eating disorders*. British Psychological Society and Gaskell, 2004.

Pike KM, Walsh BT, Vitousek K et al. Cognitive behavior therapy in the posthospitalization treatment of anorexia nervosa. *Am J Psychiatry* 2003;160:2046–9.

Shedler J. The efficacy of psychodynamic psychotherapy. *Am Psychol* 2010;65:98–109.

Zhu AJ, Walsh BT. Pharmacologic treatment of eating disorders. *Can J Psychiatry* 2002;47:227–34.

Studies of treatment options for bulimia are more advanced than those for anorexia. The focus of the majority of these studies is on young adult populations. For patients suffering from bulimia, the most common modes of treatment involve psychological therapy, medication or a combination of both. Evidence shows that treatment can be successful, but it is still unclear whether significant risks and vulnerabilities for recurrence ever completely resolve in severe cases.

Stepped care approach

The treatment for bulimia involves a stepped care approach, starting with primary care and/or self-help programs; this is followed, as necessary, by hospital outpatient or day treatment, then inpatient treatment in a general psychiatry unit or, preferably, specialist unit-based therapies.

Recent studies on the treatment of bulimia have demonstrated that, for adults, cognitive interventions and antidepressants, especially selective serotonin-reuptake inhibitors (SSRIs), are effective. These findings do not necessarily apply to adolescents. For the younger patients, family therapy may be indicated; ultimately, data indicate that intensive treatment modalities play an important role in any attempt at recovery.

The primary goals of treatment for bulimia are:
- to help a patient stop bingeing and purging
- to help a patient learn, regain and maintain healthy eating patterns
- to address other psychological issues related to the primary diagnosis of bulimia.

Non-pharmacological treatment

The most commonly used treatments for patients with bulimia are psychological and patient-led interventions. Non-pharmacological methods include:

- cognitive–behavior therapy (CBT)
- behavioral techniques
- relaxation training
- stimulus control
- family and marital therapy
- group therapy
- support groups/stepped programs
- self-help approaches.

Cognitive–behavior therapy comprises four distinct phases for patients with bulimia. Initially, a clinician makes an assessment of the patient's psychological, emotional and behavioral functioning by means of a clinical interview. The patient is also asked to self-monitor nutritional intake, and bingeing and purging behaviors. The patient is then educated about healthy regular eating patterns and is encouraged to resume or engage in nutritious eating. This is an attempt to normalize the sporadic and out-of-control dietary intake. CBT also seeks to restructure the patient's cognitive distortions about food, thinness, achievement and assertiveness. Finally, by continually discussing signs of relapse and focusing on preventative strategies, an emphasis is placed on the prevention of relapse. Therapy is slowly tapered when the patient shows consolidated signs of progress.

Behavioral techniques. The technique of exposure plus response prevention is often used, and is based on a model of anxiety and phobic avoidance that is involved in the binge–purge cycle. Patients are made to eat foods that they fear either gradually or through a binge and are then prevented from purging. Repeated exposure to the foods without compensatory purging behaviors aims to decrease the patient's anxiety over time. Concomitantly, the patient also becomes less fearful of normal eating.

Relaxation training. A prime example of relaxation training is progressive muscle relaxation. Patients with bulimia benefit from learning alternative means of dealing with negative emotions such as anxiety. Patients follow a routine of tightening and relaxing muscles in their entire body while playing a pre-planned tape of smooth calming music with narrated instructions. Relaxation training becomes increasingly useful as patients become more comfortable with the techniques and are able to maximize the benefits of the exercise.

Stimulus control. With this technique, antecedent and consequential behaviors associated with bingeing and purging are examined and restructured to prevent binges and purges.

Family and marital therapy. Patients whose family and marital dynamics contribute to, or exacerbate, bulimic symptoms may benefit from family or marital therapy. A study of 49 adolescents with eating disorders and their families found that mothers' critical comments explained 28–34% of the variance in outcome for the patients, and that it was the best predictor of outcome. Two studies of the family environments of patients with bulimia showed that punishment contributed to overall outcome difficulties and was indicative of poor family functioning.

There have been promising results in studies of adolescents with bulimia who still live with their parents. For example, a pilot study found that treatment of female patients (aged 14–17 years) with brief family therapy resulted in significant decreases in bulimic behavior at 1 year. This type of therapy has also produced good results in older patients with marital discord or ongoing conflicts with parents. However, it is generally less effective than in patients with anorexia.

Group therapy. Patients who demonstrate particularly poor social skills and who appear particularly susceptible to group or societal pressures toward thinness may benefit from group therapy targeted at bulimia recovery. This method may also help patients to deal more effectively with the feelings of shame commonly surrounding the disorder, as well as provide additional peer-based feedback and support.

Support groups/stepped programs. Some patients have found groups and programs such as Overeaters Anonymous (see page 105) to be helpful, in conjunction with initial treatments, for the prevention of relapses. These programs, however, should not be used as the primary treatment for bulimia.

Self-help approaches. There is increasing support for self-help or guided self-help manuals that can successfully deliver CBT for adults with bulimia. Using an evidence-based self-help program, with or without a trial of antidepressant drug, is proposed as the first step approach in the UK guidance issued by the National Institute for Health and Clinical Excellence (NICE). Further development of such programs may prove to be important in providing treatment to patients who otherwise would not have access to adequate care.

Interpersonal psychotherapy (IPT) emphasizes interpersonal relationships rather than eating habits or attitudes toward weight and shape. Initial sessions explore the interpersonal context within which the eating disorder has developed and has been maintained in order to identify problem areas. Subsequent sessions develop and review interpersonal changes, rather than cognitive or behavioral changes, to treat the disorder. IPT has not been systematically studied in young people.

Dialectical behavioral therapy (DBT). This method is based on the affect regulation model, which views bulimic behaviors as a means to cope with negative emotions. The goal of therapy is to equip patients with the skills to respond to the maladaptive emotions that induce binge eating and purging with adaptive behaviors, such as mindfulness and deep breathing.

Pharmacological treatment

Although the mainstay of treatment for bulimia is non-pharmacological, more research has been conducted on the pharmacological treatment of bulimia than of anorexia. Most clinicians treat bulimia with SSRIs because they are the best tolerated drugs available, with side effects that are easy to monitor.

Antidepressants have been used in the treatment of bulimia with encouraging results, and about 30% of patients benefit from pharmacotherapy alone.

Fluoxetine is commonly used for the treatment of bulimia; it is approved for use in bulimic patients in the UK and it is the only medication approved by the US Food and Drug Administration (FDA) for this eating disorder. Fluoxetine has been found to be a useful intervention for individuals with bulimia who had not responded to psychotherapy or who had relapsed after psychotherapy, producing short-term reductions in bulimic behaviors. However, more research is needed to determine the long-term effects of this drug and other antidepressants.

In general, higher doses of SSRIs are used for the treatment of bulimia than for depression, with careful monitoring of side effects. A maximum daily dosage of 60 mg can be given. Lower doses are needed in adolescents. In those, the increased risk for psychomotor activation and suicidal events potentially associated with the use of SSRIs needs to be taken into account when deciding to start or increase medication, and close monitoring is warranted throughout treatment.

Fluoxetine is contraindicated in patients taking concurrent monoamine oxidase inhibitors (MAOIs) and within 14 days of a MAOI. Care must be taken in patients with:
- renal or hepatic impairment
- a bipolar disorder
- a seizure disorder
- diabetes mellitus
- suicidal ideation.

Concomitant use of non-sedative antihistamines may carry an increased risk of arrhythmias, and the effect of anticoagulants may be enhanced.

A withdrawal syndrome is seen in up to 60% of patients in whom an SSRI other than fluoxetine is stopped suddenly. This syndrome can cause dizziness, anxiety, agitation, confusion, tremor, paresthesias, nausea and sweating. Other common side effects of SSRIs include:
- gastrointestinal reactions (nausea, vomiting, indigestion, abdominal pain, diarrhea), which are dose-related
- seizures, anxiety, fatigue, dizziness, tremor, insomnia

- antimuscarinic effects (e.g. dry mouth, constipation, urinary retention)
- sexual effects such as reduced libido, delayed ejaculation and absence of orgasms.

Tricyclic antidepressants. Although there had been initial evidence supporting the efficacy of imipramine and desipramine for bulimia, these are now considered to be an outdated treatment for bulimia. In the absence of better alternatives, doses of tricyclic antidepressants similar to those used to treat depression (150–300 mg/day) can be administered. Lower doses are needed in children and adolescents.

Imipramine should not be given to patients with a recent myocardial infarction, an arrhythmia (particularly heart block) or a seizure disorder. Imipramine and other tricyclic antidepressants should be prescribed cautiously to patients who are at risk for suicide because of the toxicity of these medications in overdose, which can be fatal. Care is also needed in patients with hepatic impairment, thyroid disease, pheochromocytoma, closed-angle glaucoma or a history of urinary retention.

The main side effects of tricyclic antidepressants include:
- dizziness, drowsiness
- tachycardia, arrhythmias, orthostatic hypotension
- anticholinergic effects (e.g. dry mouth, blurred vision, constipation, urinary retention)
- acute renal failure
- blood dyscrasias.

Imipramine should not be given within 14 days of a MAOI.

Other medications. Numerous other agents have demonstrated efficacy in the treatment of bulimia in double-blind placebo-controlled studies. These include newly indicated SSRIs such as sertraline (but not fluvoxamine) and other antidepressants such as trazodone. Bupropion is not recommended as it has been associated with seizures in purging bulimics.

Monoamine oxidase inhibitors such as phenelzine have been used for the treatment of bulimia. Doses similar to those used to treat depression can be administered. However, MAOIs are potentially dangerous to patients with chaotic bingeing and purging, so they should be administered cautiously.

Lithium carbonate, a mood stabilizer, has been used experimentally without evidence of efficacy, except in depressed bulimic patients. Its use frequently leads to undesirable weight gain; mood stabilizers that avoid this problem may prove more effective. Lithium carbonate is now used at times as an adjunct for treating comorbid conditions.

Topiramate, an antiepileptic medication with mood-stabilizing properties, has been shown to be effective for reducing binge or purge frequency. In clinical trials, it has been associated with low rates of adverse effects, but practitioners have reported side effects such as word-finding difficulties and paresthesias. These side effects may be the result of increasing doses too quickly.

Ondansetron, an antiemetic, has been shown to reduce bingeing and purging, but must be administered several times throughout the day and is expensive. It is not recommended because there are insufficient supportive data and understanding about the physiological outcomes in bulimia.

Naltrexone, an opioid antagonist, shows some efficacy at doses higher than those used for prevention of relapse from narcotic addiction and alcohol abuse, but there are some concerns regarding hepatotoxicity at high doses.

Optimizing treatment

Up to 70% of patients with bulimia benefit from a combination of medication and cognitive–behavior interventions. Studies have demonstrated that the symptoms of bingeing, purging and other attitudes related to eating disorders respond better to psychotherapy than to medication alone. A combination of the two modalities has been shown to be more effective for some outcomes than either by itself.

In one study, CBT produced better results than treatment with fluoxetine, and although a combination intervention showed some benefit, there was a high rate of attrition. In another study, intensive group cognitive psychotherapy demonstrated greater efficacy than imipramine for the treatment of bingeing, purging and the symptoms of depression. Although the combination of the treatments did not incrementally improve 'eating variables' such as fear of gaining weight, body-image distortion, bingeing and purging, it did reduce depression and anxiety.

CBT has demonstrated greater benefit than supportive psychotherapy, while sequential medication with desipramine followed by fluoxetine (a typically used regimen) was superior to placebo; a combination of CBT and sequential medication produced the highest rates of abstinence. Group CBT has also demonstrated superior efficacy to desipramine, while a combination of the two treatments demonstrated improvement in some variables such as dietary restraint.

Follow-up

Regular follow-up assessments may be beneficial to ensure that healthy eating patterns are being maintained and to assess the patient's long-term coping skills. Some patients find support groups helpful. Regular moderate exercise may help patients to deal with the weight fluctuations that can be expected while their bodies adjust to the new healthy eating patterns. Researchers in the UK suggest that, overall, readiness to change and the development of the therapeutic alliance are more strongly related to improvement than the specific type of treatment offered to patients with bulimia.

Key points – treatment of bulimia

- The main goals of treatment for bulimia are abstinence from bingeing and purging, learning and maintaining healthy eating behaviors, and addressing any other psychological issues related to the condition.
- Psychological interventions are the mainstay of treatment; symptoms of bingeing and purging and other aspects of eating disorders respond better to psychotherapy than to medication alone.
- Up to 70% of patients benefit from a combination of cognitive–behavior techniques and pharmacotherapy.
- Higher doses of selective serotonin-reuptake inhibitors are used for the treatment of bulimia than for depression, with careful monitoring of side effects.
- Fluoxetine is the only medication approved by the US Food and Drug Administration for the treatment of bulimia; it is also licensed for this use in the UK.
- Regular moderate exercise may help patients to deal with the weight fluctuations that can be expected while their bodies adjust to new healthy eating patterns.

Key references

Agras WS, Walsh T, Fairburn CG et al. A multicenter comparison of cognitive-behavioral therapy and interpersonal psychotherapy for bulimia nervosa. *Arch Gen Psychiatry* 2000;57:459–66.

Bacaltchuk J. Hay P, Trefiglio R. Antidepressants versus psychological treatments and their combination for bulimia nervosa. *Cochrane Database Syst Rev* 2001;4:CD003385.

Flament MF, Bissada H, Spettigue W. Evidence-based pharmacotherapy of eating disorders. *Int J Neuropsychopharmacol* 2011. Epub ahead of print (doi: 10.1017/S1461145711000381).

Goldbloom DS, Olmsted M, Davis R et al. A randomized controlled trial of fluoxetine and cognitive behavioral therapy for bulimia nervosa: short-term outcome. *Behav Res Ther* 1997;35:803–11.

Hedges DW, Reimherr FW, Hoopes SP et al. Treatment of bulimia nervosa with topiramate in a randomized, double-blind, placebo-controlled trial, part 2: improvement in psychiatric measures. *J Clin Psychiatry* 2003;64:1449–54.

Herzog DB, Dorer DJ, Keel PK et al. Recovery and relapse in anorexia and bulimia nervosa: a 7.5-year follow-up study. *J Am Acad Child Adolesc Psychiatry* 1999;38:829–37.

Hoopes SP, Reimherr FW, Hedges DW et al. Treatment of bulimia nervosa with topiramate in a randomized, double-blind, placebo-controlled trial, part 1: improvement in binge and purge measures. *J Clin Psychiatry* 2003;64:1335–41.

Jonas JM, Gold MS. Treatment of antidepressant-resistant bulimia with naltrexone. *Int J Psychiatry Med* 1986;16:305–9.

Safer DL, Telch CF, Agras WS. Dialectical behavior therapy for bulimia nervosa. *Am J Psychiatry* 2001;158:632–4.

Treasure JL, Katzman M, Schmidt U et al. Engagement and outcomes in the treatment of bulimia nervosa: first phase of a sequential design comparing motivation enhancement therapy and cognitive behavioural therapy. *Behav Res Ther* 1999;37:405–18.

van Furth EF, van Strien DC, Martina LM et al. Expressed emotion and the prediction of outcome in adolescent eating disorders. *Int J Eat Disord* 1996;20:19–31.

Walsh BT, Agras WS, Devlin MJ et al. Fluoxetine for bulimia nervosa following poor response to psychotherapy. *Am J Psychiatry* 2000;157:1332–4.

Anorexia

The course of anorexia is variable, with remission rates differing considerably across long-term outcome studies with follow-up periods of 1–30 years. In over 100 studies published in the second half of the 20th century, fewer than one half of anorexic patients recovered on average, whereas one-third improved, and 20% remained chronically ill. In seven studies published since 2004, most patients with anorexia ascertained through outpatient settings had achieved remission by 5-year follow-up, but inpatient samples had lower remission rates. In these most recent studies, rates of continued anorexia at follow-up ranged from 2% in a 9-year follow-up of patients at a community clinic, to 18% at 12 years for individuals from an inpatient center; other participants who did not achieve remission over the course of follow-up had moved to a diagnosis of either bulimia or eating disorder not otherwise specified (EDNOS).

One consistent finding across long-term studies has been that a large proportion of anorexic patients followed over time suffered from additional psychiatric disorders, including anxiety disorders, affective disorders, substance-use disorders, obsessive–compulsive disorder and borderline or histrionic personality disorders; schizophrenia is only rarely observed at follow-up. There seems to be a critical threshold of duration of illness (of about 12 years) after which it is increasingly unlikely that patients will recover, regardless of the interventions used. As anorexia usually begins in mid-adolescence, this puts the critical age at about 30 years.

Some researchers suggest a starvation-dependence model, likening it to alcohol dependence. Under such a hypothesis, patients are both psychologically and physiologically addicted to the effects of starvation, and persistent weight loss may reflect a tolerance for starvation. More than one-third of patients have recurrent affective illnesses. Although vocational and academic functioning may be satisfactory, psychological and social impairments often persist even after weight restoration.

In a study comparing the outcomes of patients with anorexia and bulimia, researchers found that the number of patients making a full recovery was twice as high in the group with bulimia than in the group with anorexia; approximately one-third of each group relapsed after full recovery.

Variables affecting outcome. In long-term outcome studies of anorexia nervosa, the findings regarding prognostic factors have also been very heterogeneous. Most studies indicated that a short duration of symptoms before treatment resulted in a favorable outcome, but findings are ambiguous regarding age at onset of illness. No definite conclusions could be drawn as to whether greater weight loss at presentation had long-term effects on outcome, but it is clear that vomiting, bulimia and purgative abuse imply an unfavorable prognosis. A few studies have also shown that premorbid development and clinical abnormalities, including eating disorders during childhood, have a negative prognostic significance. In contrast, a good parent–child relationship may protect the patient from a poor outcome. In addition, the data clearly show that chronicity leads to negative outcome, a finding that implies that there are cases of anorexia refractory to treatment. The features of coexisting obsessive–compulsive personality seem to add to chronicity.

A cross-cultural study revealed that the outcome of an adolescent eating disorder is relatively similar across cultures, and that a later onset leads to a better prognosis. No definite conclusion can be drawn from the outcome studies as to the relevance of socioeconomic status.

Medical complications that affect adolescents rather than adults are the potential for significant growth retardation, pubertal delay or interruption, and reduction in peak bone mass. Effects on reproductive functioning are shown in Table 8.1. Women who become pregnant should be considered to be at high risk of complications (Table 8.2) and monitored through pregnancy and postpartum. Compared with non-anorexic controls, women with anorexia are more likely to have postpartum depression, and low birth weight and feeding problems in their babies.

TABLE 8.1

Effects of anorexia on reproductive functioning

- Failure to ovulate
- Oligomenorrhea
- Amenorrhea
- Reduced sex drive
- Infertility
- Hyperemesis gravidarum

TABLE 8.2

Complications of anorexia in pregnancy

- Insufficient weight gain
- Underweight babies for gestational date
- Higher frequency of cesarean section births
- Low birthweight infants
- Increased congenital anomalies
- Increased neonatal morbidity
- Problems in infant feeding

Mortality. Anorexia has the highest mortality rate of any psychological disorder. Risk of death because of complications of anorexia is 6–15%, with half the deaths resulting from suicide. In a prospective 21-year follow-up study, 16% of 84 patients with anorexia had died from the disorder and its complications. Across studies published since 2004, the crude mortality rates have ranged from 0 to 8%, with a cumulative rate of 2.8%. These rates are lower than those previously reported, which may reflect improvement in medical stabilization of the patients and/or study recruitment from sources with less severely ill cases.

Bulimia

As previously discussed, onset of bulimia usually occurs during late adolescence and early adulthood. Binge eating generally begins during an episode of restricted eating and prolonged dieting. If identified at this early stage, patients typically seek treatment and appear to be motivated to overcome the problem. However, once the act of purging starts and is reinforced, patients become extremely resistant to changing their habits. Without treatment most patients experience a chronic fluctuation of binge/purge behavior. Although individuals with bulimia experience variations in their weight, they rarely approach the low weight ranges associated with anorexia.

Recent data are available on the longitudinal course of bulimia from a total of 79 study series covering over 5000 patients followed between 6 months and 12 years. On average, close to 45% of the patients showed full recovery from bulimia, whereas 27% improved considerably, and nearly 23% had a chronic protracted course. Crossover to another eating disorder (most often EDNOS, more rarely anorexia) at the follow-up evaluation amounted to a mean of 22.5%. The data suggest a curvilinear course, with highest recovery rates between 4 and 9 years of follow-up, and reverse peaks for both improvement and chronicity before 4 years and after 10 years of follow-up. Although many studies have investigated potential prognostic factors, there was only conflicting evidence.

As stated above, the course and outcome for women with bulimia is generally more favorable than for those with anorexia. A study in the UK found that bulimia and binge-eating disorder among young women had different courses and outcomes. While the prognosis of those with bulimia was relatively poor, the majority of those with binge-eating disorder recovered during a 5-year follow-up period.

Medical complications include hypokalemia and other electrolyte imbalances, esophageal tears, gastric disturbances, dehydration and orthostatic blood-pressure changes, which may lead to intermittent hospitalization.

Mortality. Across outcome studies of bulimia, crude mortality rates have ranged from 0 to 2%, with a cumulative mortality rate of 0.4%. Adjusting for duration of follow-up, death appeared to be five times less likely to occur in bulimia than in anorexia across the studies reviewed.

Key points – course and prognosis

- Despite increasing research on short- and long-term outcomes of anorexia, the disease still has a relatively poor prognosis; the mortality rate is the highest of all psychiatric disorders, although it has decreased in recent years.
- Although results from long-term studies support optimism for most patients with eating disorders, approximately 30% of patients with bulimia and atypical eating disorders remain ill at 10–20 years following presentation.
- Anorexia can have serious effects on reproductive functioning and the health of neonates.
- Bulimia usually persists for several years, and associated medical complications can result in intermittent hospitalization.

Key references

Fairburn CG, Cooper Z, Doll HA et al. The natural course of bulimia nervosa and binge eating disorder in young women. *Arch Gen Psychiatry* 2000;57:659–65.

Keel PK, Brown TA. Update on course and outcome in eating disorder. *Int J Eat Disord* 2010;43:195–204.

Mitchell JE, Crow S. Medical complications of anorexia nervosa and bulimia nervosa. *Curr Opin Psychiatry* 2006;19:438–43.

Steinhausen HC. The outcome of anorexia nervosa in the 20th century. *Am J Psychiatry* 2002;159:1284–93.

Steinhausen HC, Boyadjieva S, Grigoroiu-Serbanescu M et al. A transcultural outcome study of adolescent eating disorders. *Acta Psychiatr Scand* 2000;101:60–6.

Steinhausen HC, Weber S. The outcome of bulimia nervosa: findings from one-quarter century of research. *Am J Psychiatry* 2009;166:1331–41.

Eating disorders not otherwise specified

As mentioned in Chapter 1, the classification of 'eating disorders not otherwise specified' (EDNOS), the third diagnostic category of eating disorders in the American Psychiatric Association's *Diagnostic and Statistical Manual of Mental Disorders* Fourth Edition (DSM-IV), is given to cases that do not fulfill the full criteria for anorexia or bulimia, and is the most frequently given diagnosis for eating disorders. Examples of EDNOS diagnoses are:

- female patients who meet all the criteria for anorexia yet menstruate regularly
- individuals who meet all the criteria for anorexia but despite significant weight loss maintain weight in the normal range
- individuals who display combinations of binge eating and inappropriate compensatory behaviors but at lower frequencies than those stipulated in the criteria.

EDNOS also includes two subsets of disorders that have been defined by specific diagnostic criteria and have received increasing research interest: binge-eating disorder (BED) and night-eating syndrome (NES).

Binge-eating disorder, or non-purging bulimia, is characterized as recurrent episodes of binge eating, accompanied by a sense of distress, and feelings of disgust, depression or guilt, without the subsequent inappropriate compensatory behaviors (purging or non-purging) associated with bulimia. Hence, BED is often associated with overweight or obesity. There is increasing consent in the literature to consider BED as its own diagnostic category because of its distinct features, treatment and prognosis compared with bulimia. The overall prevalence of BED has been estimated as 3.5% in women and 2.0% in men. Compared with anorexia and bulimia, the sex ratio is less uneven, with males making up about 40–50% of EDNOS diagnoses with a BED subcategory. Age of onset for BED is slightly higher than for bulimia, ranging from 17 to 32 years, with a mean of 25 years. BED has an overall better prognosis than bulimia, however, as it responds to a wider range of treatments that target both binge eating and weight reduction. Although the types of treatment are the same as those used for patients with bulimia, BED is more responsive to various subtypes of treatment such as medication and CBT.

CBT and interpersonal therapy (IPT) have appeared equally effective in reducing binge eating, although they do not lead to clinically significant weight loss. Pharmacotherapy has used anticonvulsant agents such as topiramate, which have been associated with a reduction in both binge eating and weight. In one study, the combination of topiramate and CBT led to an abstinence rate of 80% compared with 61% for placebo. The selective serotonin-reuptake inhibitors (SSRIs), including fluvoxamine, sertraline, fluoxetine, citalopram and escitalopram, as well as the antiobesity medication sibutramine, all have appeared superior to placebo for reduction in binge frequency, weight loss and improvement of general illness severity, although long-term studies are still lacking.

Night-eating syndrome is characterized by insomnia, excessive appetite (hyperphagia) in the evening and a lack of appetite in the morning. Individuals with NES wake several times throughout the night to eat, consuming over a third of their total energy intake after their evening meal. Binge eating or purging behaviors are generally not associated with this disorder, and these individuals can usually recall what they ate. In contrast, nocturnal eating/drinking syndrome is characterized by recurrent episodes of binge eating throughout the night with no, or partial, recollection of what was eaten. This syndrome is a combination of an eating, sleep and mood disorder. Limited research has been conducted on effective treatments for NES, but the SSRI sertraline has shown some benefit.

Feeding disorders

In young children, problems with eating are called feeding disorders. These disorders are believed to reflect the relationship between parent and child, as opposed to just the child or the adolescent as is the case with eating disorders. There is no extensive literature on this subject, but the typical dyad seems to be a single, young, socially isolated, anxious mother with a difficult infant.

There are three DSM-IV categories of feeding disorders: feeding disorder of infancy and early childhood; rumination disorder; and pica.

Feeding disorder of infancy and early childhood is a problem with feeding such that a child does not eat properly, resulting in weight loss or inability to gain adequate weight. This problem must first present under 6 years of age to meet the diagnostic criteria.

Rumination disorder is the regurgitation and rechewing of food in an infant or child and presents after a period of normal functioning. Onset is usually between 3 and 12 months of age.

Pica is the repeated eating of non-nutritive substances such as paint, plaster, string, hair or cloth. This problem usually presents in infancy and remits in early childhood. Pica is associated with pervasive developmental disorder and mental retardation.

Diagnosis and management. Feeding disorder diagnoses are only given if symptoms last for at least 1 month, cannot be explained by other medical problems and are severe enough to warrant independent clinical attention. Treatment includes medical interventions for malnutrition and behavioral interventions to build healthy feeding patterns.

Key points – other eating disorders

- Eating disorders not otherwise specified is the category of diagnosis given to cases that do not fulfill all DSM-IV criteria for anorexia or bulimia; subtypes of this category include binge-eating disorder (BED) and night-eating syndrome (NES).
- There is a higher prevalence of BED than anorexia or bulimia in men.
- The peak age of onset for BED is somewhat later than that for bulimia, and BED has an overall better prognosis.
- Individuals with NES wake several times throughout the night to eat, consuming over one-third of their total energy intake after their evening meal.
- Feeding disorders in young children are categorized as feeding disorder of infancy and childhood, rumination disorder or pica.

Key references

American Psychiatric Association. Eating disorders. *Diagnostic and Statistical Manual of Mental Disorders*, 4th edn. Text Revision (DSM-IV-TR). Washington, DC: American Psychiatric Association, 2000:589–94.

American Psychiatric Association. *Practice Guidelines for the Treatment of Psychiatric Disorders, Compendium 2006; Eating Disorders*, 3rd edn. Washington, DC: American Psychiatric Association, 2006.

Anderson CA, Lock J. Feeding disorders. In: Steiner H, Yalom ID, eds. *Treating Preschool Children*. San Francisco: Jossey-Bass, 1997: 187–207.

Flament MF, Bissada H, Spettigue W. Evidence-based pharmacotherapy of eating disorders. *Int J Neuropsychopharmacol* 2011. Epub ahead of print (doi: 10.1017/S1461145711000381)

Hudson JI, Hiripi E, Pope HG, Jr., Kessler RC. The prevalence and correlates of eating disorders in the National Comorbidity Survey Replication. *Biol Psychiatry* 2007;61:348–58.

Steiner H. Appetite disturbances: anorexia and hyperphagia. In: Noshpitz JD, ed. *Handbook of Child and Adolescent Psychiatry: Volume 5: Clinical Assessment and Intervention Planning*. New York: John Wiley and Sons, 1998:105–9.

Stunkard AJ, Allison KC. Two forms of disordered eating in obesity: binge eating and night eating. *Int J Obesity* 2003;27:1–12.

Wonderlich SA, Gordon KH, Mitchell JE et al. The validity and clinical utility of binge eating disorder. *Int J Eat Disord* 2009;42:687–705.

Developmental studies

Eating disorders are often conceptualized as developmental disorders, but only a few studies have approached eating disorders from a developmental perspective and the data are limited. Research is needed to determine the factors that result in risk or resilience to the development of an eating disorder during specific times in a child's development.

Treatment outcome studies – particularly those applying standardized screening instruments – were rare 10 years ago; clearly this has changed. However, some design problems persist: while most studies involve mixed populations of juveniles and adults they rarely control for age of onset of illness and duration of illness, thus confounding results. Studies addressing these issues from a developmental perspective need to be conducted. This may require treatment to be tailored to developmental stage.

Additional randomized controlled clinical trials, sophisticated multicenter comparisons, and studies investigating the long-term efficacy of different psychotherapies and psychopharmacological interventions all need to be undertaken.

Genetic studies

Hypotheses on the etiology of bulimia have spanned the gamut of possibilities. From familial to organic to psychosocial factors, researchers have come to realize that a combination of several factors is often responsible for the development of bulimia. Promising areas of future investigation include studies on genetic predisposition to anorexia and bulimia.

Studies on candidate genes have mainly focused on the serotonergic system and on genes involved in bodyweight regulation. Efforts are being focused on the A allele of the serotonin transporter gene (*HTR2A*) and a possible role in the predisposition to anorexia.

Psyche or soma?

Other avenues of future investigation hope to determine whether bulimia is an issue of psyche or soma. Researchers from Maudsley Hospital, London, UK, have emphasized the complex interaction between biological and psychological factors leading to a lifestyle of bingeing and purging. Future studies that identify the interplay between organic and psychosocial causation are under way. As many scientists believe, focusing exclusively on either aspect would be a disservice to bulimic patients everywhere.

Case A – typical young woman with anorexia nervosa

This Asian-American patient presented at age 15. She had been referred by her pediatrician who had unsuccessfully attempted to halt her steady weight loss for the past 12 months by tracking her weight weekly and having the patient consult with a dietitian. The patient was referred for vital sign instability and severe malnutrition due to progressive restriction of energy intake. Her instability was such that she was immediately hospitalized in our comprehensive care unit to receive concomitant pediatric and psychiatric care. There was no associated purging or laxative or diet pill abuse. She had achieved a 40 pound weight loss by energy restriction down to 600 calories a day and increased caloric expenditure (daily exercise of up to 2 hours, aerobic and anaerobic). She fulfilled all the diagnostic criteria for anorexia nervosa (weight loss of almost 30% from her initial weight, where she had a BMI of 24.2; a continued desire to lose weight, with a strong belief that she still was overweight; and cessation of menses for 5 months).

The illness began shortly after her father had returned to the parental home after a 4-year absence. The parents had separated but had not apprised the rest of the family of this fact. The two eldest of the six children in the family had been told that father and mother had marital difficulties; the four youngest ones, among them the patient, were told that the father was on a long business trip in Asia. The patient reported that she had awakened one day to find her father gone, then 4 years later he reappeared without there being any detailed explanation of his absence. The patient, the fourth of the children, had an especially close relationship to her father, much closer than to her mother. Any inquiry on her part was met with the counter that children should not ask so many questions. Upon his return, the father commented on the fact that the patient "had really filled out and should watch her diet a bit more".

During the year before hospitalization, the pediatrician had first worked up other possible causes for weight loss, but all tests of gastrointestinal functioning and metabolic status were within normal limits, other than the indications of secondary manifestations of semi-starvation. Attempts to refer the family for a psychiatric consultation were met with resistance on the part of the patient, and her family did not insist effectively on completing this part of the evaluation, associating psychiatric care with stigma and shame, and attempting to preserve the cover up of the father's unexplained absence.

An exploration of the patient's background and developmental history revealed that several family members (first and second degree) had problems with anxiety-related symptoms: her mother had obsessive shopping for groceries, several times a day; a younger sister had pronounced separation anxiety; and a maternal grandmother described classic panic attacks. All these were undiagnosed and untreated. On the father's side there was a history of compulsive gambling (father and grandfather). One older sister had gone through a period of unexplained profound weight loss during puberty, but this was never diagnosed and treated, and resolved with her moving away to college. The relationship of this older sister with the family was tenuous.

The patient's development was characterized by pronounced separation anxiety and trouble with transition into school; the complete absence of camp experiences and sleepovers; and a limited circle of social extrafamilial peer contacts. The patient's mother reported fussy eating and rigid circadian rhythms from a very early age on. There were no traumatic events up until the father's prolonged absence; pubertal development coincided with the father's exit from the family and was not handled well in the chaos ensuing in the family. The patient was not given any helpful detail regarding the implications of her bodily changes. There was no dating history: the family's expectation was that any such activity would be delayed until the girl's twenties and would be closely linked to being on her way to becoming married. Premarital sex was explicitly forbidden.

The family valued academic success highly, and there was considerable pressure to follow the older siblings' footsteps (one was a lawyer, the other a doctor, having graduated from elite academic institutions). The family also placed great emphasis on extracurricular achievements. The patient had dedicated most of her spare time to ballet. She was quite successful up until early adolescence, when following menarche, she began to develop into a more full-figured young woman. There was considerable pressure from her teachers to lose weight. Ballet had a special significance to the patient, as her father had taken special pleasure in her dance success and she diligently attempted to continue her prepubertal trajectory, despite the fact that this became increasingly difficult to combine with her gain in weight and stature.

Examining her preferred ways of handling stress, her profile revealed avoidant coping and immature ways of reacting to the unexpected, manifesting in withdrawal, magical thinking, ritualistic behavior and extreme altruism.

The patient's treatment included a standardized nutritional rehabilitation program under the direction of the pediatric team, with: active daily dietary consultation; individual psychiatric sessions aimed at establishing a working alliance and at a more detailed exploration of her emotional reactions to her pubertal changes; twice-weekly family therapy sessions with the father and mother aimed at the exploration of latent conflict and the clarification of family secrets; and daily group therapy sessions aimed at the patient's re-education of her understanding of pubertal development, nutrition, eating behaviors and weight gain.

The patient was evaluated for use of psychopharmacological agents, but as her nutritional status was so poor and her emotional status subdued because of the effects of her pronounced malnutrition, it was decided to re-evaluate the need for targeted medication treatment of anxiety as her weight gain progressed. Her discharge weight was set at 80% of ideal bodyweight so as to maximize her chances of completing her treatment as an outpatient.

The initial 3 weeks of weight and nutritional rehabilitation proceeded uneventfully. The patient gained at the regular pace of 2–3 pounds a week and her vital signs began to improve. In individual sessions she presented as a sweet compliant woman with great reluctance to look at the significance of her symptoms beyond her fear of being obese and her desire to lose weight. Family sessions resulted in the parents revealing to the rest of the family the true background to the father's absence, paired with reassurances that their marriage was on the mend and there were no further plans to separate. Also absent was any appreciation of how difficult the past 4 years would have been for the patient, or any apologies for how the situation was handled. The argument used repeatedly was, "Look, it did not affect any of the other kids, so why should this be so important to the patient," ignoring the patient's special close ties with her father.

As the patient's weight approached the projected 80% ideal bodyweight, several changes were notable. She became more emotional and visibly anxious around meal time. She exhibited several compensatory behaviors which signaled increasing non-compliance – cutting food into small pieces, hiding food, complaining about portion sizes and debating the necessity for further weight gain. The parents interpreted that as the treatment team's inability to treat her anorexia properly and started questioning the need for further hospitalization. This also coincided with the family sessions taking on increasing intensity, as the parents were asked to take over monitoring the patient's intake and to help her with eating. The family sessions also left some doubt as to whether the marital conflict was truly resolved. As soon as the patients' vital signs had stabilized, the patient begged the parents to take her home, promising them continued weight gain and compliance. Another source of pressure was the girl's absence from school, with everyone concerned about her academic progress. All this coalesced into the parents removing the patient from the hospital at 75% ideal bodyweight.

After two outpatient clinic visits, the parents transferred care back to their primary care doctor. They stopped all psychiatric follow-up care. This resulted in relapse within a month following discharge from the hospital. The weight loss was not as pronounced as on first admission. The father had also gone again, back to Asia, and in the course of this hospitalization it became clear that he had a second family in Mumbai and had no further intention to return to the US family. As family sessions had inched closer to revealing this, the family had decided to break off treatment the first time around.

The second round of weight rehabilitation was more extended, and characterized by symptoms of grieving and depression in the mother as well as the patient. Now that the father was not present, the older siblings – particularly the older sister – became more effectively involved in the treatment. The older sister was extremely helpful in moving psychotherapy along, bringing in useful discussions of the topics related to the role of women in the family while providing an excellent role model to her younger sister and a source of support for the mother. This second hospitalization also effectively terminated any further involvement in ballet, providing a face-saving excuse for the patient to discontinue an activity which would not give her any further pleasure and provided several challenges to her medical stability.

Following hospitalization, the patient and her family remained in treatment for the next 2.5 years. Family sessions were completed after about 20 sessions and after the patient had become able to monitor her own energy intake and weight effectively with some pediatric/nutritional consultation. The patient remained in individual therapy until after her completion of high school. She was accepted into an elite college on the East Coast, necessitating her separation from the family. This posed some problems with anxiety on her and her mother's part, but these resolved without medication and closer monitoring of intake and weight at the receiving college. She continued checking in with her psychiatrist during school holidays for the next 2 years, but ongoing treatment was not necessary. With entry into college, she began cautiously to date, checking in with her older sister repeatedly about her partner choices.

On follow up, 3 years after conclusion of treatment, she reports that she has graduated from college and has been accepted into a doctoral psychology program back on the West Coast. She intends to pursue as her main area of interest the study of self-regulation and its relationship to the role of women. She has a steady boyfriend from the same ethnic group and they are planning to continue their relationship in graduate school. He has been accepted to medical school in the same town as she will be in, but at another college.

Case B – typical young woman with bulimia

This is the case of a 17-year-old white female junior in high school. She was referred by her pediatrician for psychiatric evaluation following the doctor's discovery that the girl had been attempting to lose weight for the past 2 years by intermittent dieting and abusing laxatives, diuretics and stimulants to control her appetite. The girl had requested this referral as she felt increasingly out of control of her eating, appetite and, in fact, her life. While she had been able to keep her throwing-up a secret for quite a long time, she was becoming increasingly frightened by the violence of her symptoms and ashamed of the self-abusive patterns of eating necessary to achieve even a modicum of stability.

The girl's problems had begun approximately 2 years previously, when her soccer coach demanded that she lose weight in order to retain her position as a starting midfielder on the school's varsity team. As the girl was hoping to go to college on a soccer stipend, she took seriously his threats that he would bench her should she not return in the Fall 25 pounds lighter. She was, in fact, only approximately 15 pounds overweight. Her weight gain ensued after she began several crash diets aimed at reducing her weight. As she was embarking on a near-starvation diet to lose weight in the summer, she found that she could not tolerate prolonged time spans without eating. She developed breakthrough eating, which could easily be categorized as bingeing (eating 3000 calories or more in less than 30 minutes). While this initially occurred only once every few weeks, by the time of referral she had developed patterns of overeating 3–5 times a week.

She tried various ways of controlling her appetite – using diuretics, laxatives, diet pills and, finally, stimulants. She had easy access to street drugs, as both of her older brothers had a history of drug abuse and selling substances to support their habit. All these efforts did not successfully reduce her weight for any length of time nor did they control her appetite, which became increasingly unpredictable and out of control. She found that the only way to prevent further weight gain somewhat successfully was through self-induced purging after each meal. At the time of referral, she found it unnecessary to actively induce vomiting; she in fact could vomit at will either leaning over the toilet or by simply pushing on her stomach forcefully. As she became more and more involved in chaotic dietary practices, her grades began to slip and she was unable to keep her spot on the varsity team. At that time she became sexually active with multiple casual partners. She used protection intermittently, but never became pregnant or had a diagnosed sexually transmitted disease.

Throughout her difficulties, the girl had retained her regular menstrual periods. Her weight never dropped more than 10 pounds maximum. She reported increasing problems with irritability, concentration, falling asleep and staying asleep and increased test anxiety. The family reported increasing non-compliance with family rules, such as curfews, and open conflict.

The girl came from a middle-class background. Her father was a college graduate who ran a cleaning business. Her mother was a high-school graduate who worked as an administrative assistant. On the father's side there was a significant history in his father of alcohol addiction, leading to him being a complete teetotaler. On the mother's side there was a significant history of depression – she was treated for prolonged postpartum depression after the birth of each of her boys. As she was now entering menopause, she reported increasing mood dysregulation. Her father was diagnosed with bipolar illness, treated with lithium, and committed suicide when she was 20.

In her psychiatric examination, the patient reported several incidents related to her drug use and sexual activity that had been quite traumatic. At one point, one of her brother's friends who was supplying her with stimulants, demanded that they have sex in lieu of payment. He became increasingly threatening towards the patient, until she finally agreed to have intercourse. She had not disclosed this episode to another person, and it was reported to child protection services in the course of the evaluation. There were several other instances where she found herself drunk at a party and was unable to remember details of what had happened. Sometimes her clothes were in disarray when she woke.

She reported that most of her episodes of overeating and subsequent purging were induced by intense emotional conflict with either her parents or boyfriends. She found that initially binge/purge cycles would help her settle down. But as her bulimia became more chronic and solidly established, she found that episodes were occurring more regularly at the end of the day, were less tied to precipitants, and without the initially calming effect she had found so useful.

As the findings were presented to the patient and the family, once again profound conflict erupted. Her father left the session in a huff, declaring he wanted nothing to do with any of this. He did not condone any of the patient's activities and was unwilling to participate in her further care. Her mother declared that she was exhausted from having to deal with her two older sons' substance abuse and tired of mediating the constant conflict between patient and father. This had a profoundly saddening effect on the patient, who became acutely suicidal and had to be hospitalized.

In hospital, the pediatric/psychiatric treatment team reiterated the findings: primary diagnosis of bulimia with secondary substance abuse. The recommended treatment was a trial of: cognitive behavioral treatment combined with a selective serotonin-reuptake inhibitor (SSRI); nutritional consultation; and pediatric supervision of weight and vital sign stability. In light of the high degree of family conflict and refusal to participate in the patient's care, family therapy, which is usually part of the standardized intervention, was not pursued. The parents were told that should they find themselves able to participate in the future, the team would welcome them to do so.

The patient made a very good working alliance with her individual therapist who began the standard cognitive behavioral therapy (CBT) program while the patient was still in hospital. The first target was the elimination of purging; weight was controlled by frequent small meals. Particularly challenging foods were initially avoided and only introduced as the patient remained abstinent from purging. All street drugs were eliminated and potential abuse was monitored through random urine drug screens. An SSRI was titrated up to therapeutic doses and maintained at that level. In this initial treatment phase the patient's experience in elite sports came to her rescue, as she found it relatively easy to follow the CBT program.

This package led to stabilization of eating and a 6-week period of complete abstinence from purging. Weight remained an issue, as the patient found it very frustrating and challenging to eat as little as 1500 calories a day and not see any drop in weight towards the agreed target.

The following year as an outpatient remained quite challenging for patient and treatment team alike. As the patient reintegrated with her family and her old drug-abusing circle of friends, her exposure to conflict and temptation intensified, as did her disappointment and grief, as she was not readmitted to the varsity team. This led to several relapses in terms of binge/purging, induced mostly by disappointing and/or upsetting events. These also led, on several occasions, to her discontinuing her SSRI treatment and once again seeking to control appetite and mood with street drugs. The ensuing weeks were characterized by repeated resolve to return to treatment and relapses mostly manifesting in recurrence of binge/purging.

It was only after the patient was accepted into a state university with on-campus housing that her remission became more stable and prolonged. She became academically very successful, developed a new circle of friends who were more interested in academic achievement than drugs, alcohol or sports. On 3-year follow up, she has remained binge/purge-free for over a year, has not had any exposure to street drugs and is an honor roll student with plans to go on to graduate school in social work. She has had several short and non-injurious relationships with boys without any firm plans to date exclusively. In the long run, she would like a family and children, but for the moment, her main focus has remained on her career development. Her relationship with her family has been somewhat distant and reserved. The mother has been able to be more involved and supportive, while the father has remained staunchly withdrawn and unsupportive.

The patient has developed a very detailed knowledge of her vulnerabilities in terms of mood, eating, starvation and street drugs, and has a realistic rescue plan for how to handle upcoming stressful events. Her weight is at the upper range of normal. She has once again become very active physically: in addition to playing casual soccer games with friends and acquaintances, she has become an avid cyclist. She trains vigorously and regularly, and participates in street races.

Useful resources

Below is a list of online resources where you can find more information on eating disorders' research and treatment, as well as support groups. Please note that, along with helpful websites, there are also sites on the Internet that advocate eating disorders. It is important that patients avoid these dangerous sites that promote the unhealthy maintenance of eating-disorder behaviors.

UK
beat
Adult helpline: 0845 634 1414
Youth helpline: 0845 634 7650
www.b-eat.co.uk

National Centre for Eating Disorders
Tel: 0854 838 2040
www.eating-disorders.org.uk

Overeaters Anonymous
Tel: 07000 784985
www.oagb.org.uk

USA
Academy for Eating Disorders
Tel: +1 847 498 4274
www.aedweb.org

American Academy of Child and Adolescent Psychiatry
Tel: +1 202 966 7300
www.aacap.org/cs/root/facts_for_fa milies/teenagers_with_eating_disord ers

Eating Disorders Coalition for Research, Policy & Action
Tel: +1 202 543 9570
www.eatingdisorderscoalition.org

Eating Disorders Research Society
www.edresearchsociety.org

National Eating Disorders Association
Helpline: 1 800 931 2237
www.nationaleatingdisorders.org

International
Australia and New Zealand Academy for Eating Disorders
Tel (Australia): +61 (0)2 8007 6875
Tel (New Zealand): +64 (0)9 887 0552
www.anzaed.org.au

National Eating Disorder Information Centre (Canada)
Toll-free: 1 866 633 4220
Tel: +1 416 340 4156
www.nedic.ca

Index

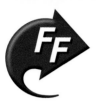

Fast Facts – the ultimate medical handbook series covers over 60 topics, including:

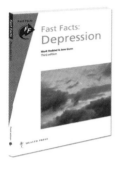

Fast Facts:
Depression
Mark Haddad & Jane Gunn
Third edition

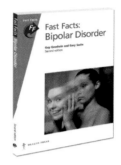

Fast Facts:
Obesity
David Haslam and Gary Wittert

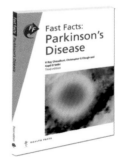

Fast Facts:
Bipolar Disorder
Guy Goodwin and Gary Sachs
Second edition

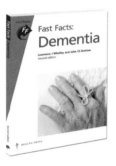

Fast Facts:
Dementia
Lawrence J Whalley and John CS Breitner
Second edition

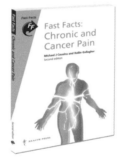

Fast Facts:
Chronic and Cancer Pain
Michael J Cousins and Kabir Gallagher
Second edition

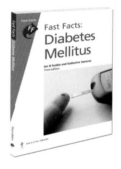

Fast Facts:
Diabetes Mellitus
Ian N Scobie and Katherine Samaras
Third edition

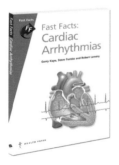

Fast Facts:
Cardiac Arrhythmias
Gerry Kaye, Steve Furniss and Robert Lemery

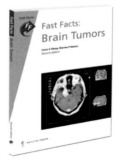

Fast Facts:
Brain Tumors
Laura E Abrey, Warren P Mason
Second edition

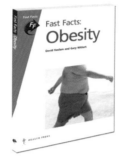

Fast Facts:
Parkinson's Disease
K Ray Chaudhuri, Christopher G Clough and Kapil D Sethi
Third edition

www.fastfacts.com

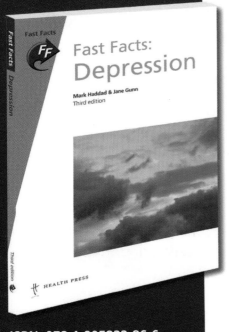

ISBN: 978-1-905832-86-6
Price: £15 • US$25 • €18

Authored by world experts...

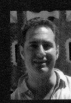

Mark Haddad PhD
RGN RMN, Clinical
Research Fellow, Institute
of Psychiatry at King's
College London, UK

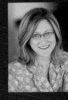

Jane Gunn PhD MBBS
DRANZCOG FRACGP
Chair, Primary Care
Research Head,
Department of General
Practice, Melbourne
Medical School,
University of Melbourne,
Australia

Fast Facts: Depression
Third edition

See below for details of how to claim your exclusive 20% discount

There are few medical handbooks that provide such a comprehensive and practical overview of current knowledge in this field. *Fast Facts: Depression* is suitable for healthcare professionals working in both primary care and specialist medical centers. It provides a depth of content that is ideal for anyone who wants to better understand depression as both an international public health problem and a common clinical mental health disorder.

3 easy steps to ordering Fast Facts books with your 20% discount

1. Visit www.fastfacts.com and add any books to your cart
2. Proceed to checkout
3. Put ED20 into the discount code box and hit apply

Visit **www.fastfacts.com** for more information, to view sample content and to place your order

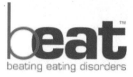

Beat is the UK's only nationwide organisation supporting people affected by eating disorders and campaigning on their behalf.

Beat's vision is that eating disorders will be beaten.

Our mission is:
- To change the way everyone thinks and talks about eating disorders
- To improve the way services and treatments are provided
- And to help anyone believe that their eating disorder can be beaten

We do this by:
- Challenging the stigma that people with eating disorders face
- Campaigning for better services and treatment
- Providing information, support and encouragement to seek recovery

Beat – beating eating disorders is a manifesto, a call to action and a message of hope.

Our activities are designed to increase knowledge, awareness and understanding of eating disorders; to provide support, help and information to people directly affected; and to increase the understanding and skills of professional staff.

We run telephone help-lines; local support groups; and a website at **www.b-eat.co.uk** with information, message boards and on-line chat. We have direct contact with individuals, and many, many thousands more through our website and the media.

We collaborate with researchers, recruiting participants for studies and trials and help disseminate research findings.

We provide training and professional development for staff in health, education and social care fields and run a biennial international conference: EDIC www.edic.org.uk.

Fast Facts, *the ultimate medical handbook series,* is now available in more formats than ever...

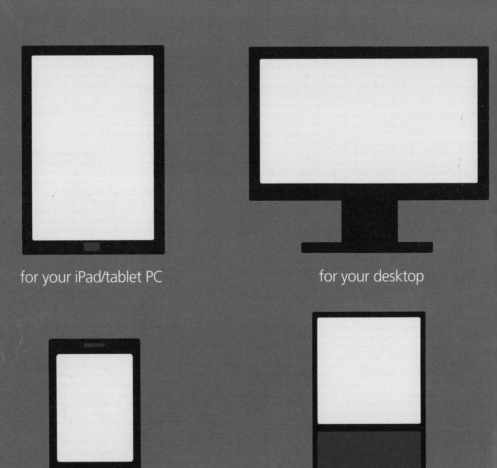

for your iPad/tablet PC

for your desktop

for your smartphone

for your eReader

eBook – compatible with any dedicated eReader
Kindle – compatible with the Kindle eReader
Mobile app – compatible with the iPhone or iPad

Visit **www.fastfacts.com** for easy ordering and special offers